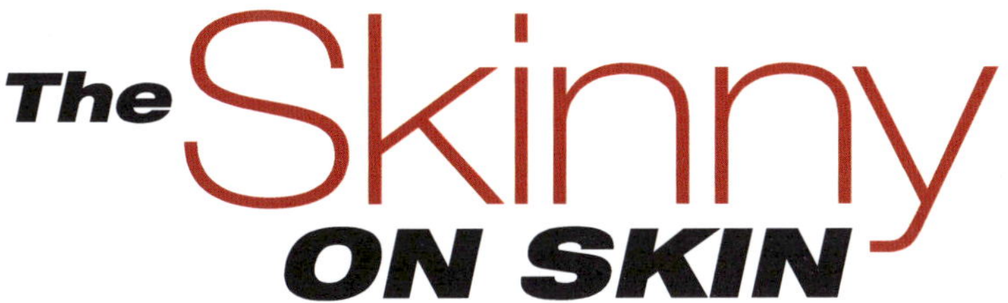

The Skinny ON SKIN

**An illustrated dermatology guide
for the public and beginning practitioners**

David James Najarian, M.D.

ISBN: 1461137179
ISBN 13: 9781461137177
Library of Congress Control Number: 2011907001
CreateSpace, North Charleston, South Carolina

Contents

Part I
Medical Skin Conditions

The Skinny on Skin

Part IV
Surgical and Other Treatments and Tests

Preface

Scientia potentia est, meaning "knowledge is power," is a Latin phrase attributed to the English philosopher Francis Bacon. It is also the theme of this book. I wrote this book with the goal of sharing my knowledge about skin with you. My hope is that this knowledge empowers you with the ability to better understand and care for skin—your own or someone else's.

FOR THE PUBLIC

If you purchased this book, you're probably looking for answers about a skin issue that you haven't found elsewhere. As a practicing dermatologist, I've had lots of patients tell me that their prior skin doctor would spend only a few minutes in the exam room with them. In those few minutes, doctors often speak quickly and use technical terms, making it difficult for patients to recall exactly what was said.

However, this is often vital information. We, as doctors, are asking you to place serious medicines in your body or on your skin. If you go home and can't remember all the reasons we thought it was important to take that medicine, you're less likely to fill that prescription. Even if you do fill the prescription, you may not recall exactly how to use the medicine. You may even forget the important side effects we said to look out for—or how to surmount them if they arise. None of this is your fault, but it's a by-product of the modern office visit. There is so much complex information that needs to be digested during a brief office session.

I understand this problem firsthand. As an acne patient in high school, I ultimately gave up on treatment because the creams were drying out my skin and not making the acne go away. If only

I had been provided with a clearer explanation for how to avoid the side effects of my creams or more effective treatment options, my problem might have been solved. Instead my acne followed me all the way to medical school and was bad enough that my advisor thought I needed to clear up my skin before applying for a dermatology residency position. One day he brought me into the room with the samples and tossed about four medications into a bag, hastily telling me how to use everything. Even as a medical student, I couldn't comprehend everything he said, and I was afraid to ask for clearer explanations. I decided, "To heck with it, I'm just going to let this go," and my acne followed me all the way to my interview sessions for dermatology residency positions. Fortunately, my true passion for skin must have shown through, because I earned a spot at my first choice—the University of Medicine and Dentistry in New Brunswick, New Jersey, near my hometown.

For all these reasons, I spent my first years in dermatology practice writing educational handouts about skin conditions to present to my patients. I still use these essays to help my patients understand what condition they have, what treatments are available to them, how to implement these treatments, and what they can expect in the future based upon the therapies they pursue. Each essay includes answers to the most common questions that arise during patient visits. Much of the medical jargon is stripped out to make the information easy to understand.

My patients take the essays home so they always have a summary of what we discussed during their visit. Many of them are happily surprised to receive this information; I have received so much positive feedback that I was inspired to mold the collection of essays into a book. Why not share this information with patients everywhere?

The book is divided into four parts. Part I explains the most common skin conditions—what causes them, how to recognize them, and how they are managed. Part II focuses on frequently prescribed medical treatments. Part III discusses cosmetic treatments, and Part IV describes surgical and other treatments and tests.

If you have a skin condition but aren't sure what you have, you can try to identify it using the table on page xv-xviii. This table is only a starting point and is limited in many ways. The only true way to arrive at a correct diagnosis is to see a dermatologist.

Keep in mind that many of the treatments discussed in this book are available over the counter without a prescription. You may find them at a pharmacy or in our online store at www. randolphdermatology.com.

FOR BEGINNING PRACTITIONERS

Dermatologists are not the only ones out there providing great skin care. We frequently team up with physician extenders, nurses, medical students, and aestheticians to help treat patients. The educational resources available to them are exhaustive—you should see the size of some of the classic dermatology textbooks! Unfortunately, many of them would take me a year or longer to read—and I'm already a board-certified dermatologist. There is so much detail in these books that one can truly get lost in the trees and lose track of the forest.

This book can be used by beginning practitioners without much spare time who need to learn the field quickly. Each essay provides critical information you need to know about the condition itself, available treatments, how to implement the treatments, and what can be anticipated from the therapies. The articles provide answers to questions patients are going to ask. Each is crafted for quick comprehension and omits details that can be found in other resources. Do not use this book to review for tests, though; it is strictly meant for patient-care issues and is written in nontechnical language that patients can easily understand.

Disclaimer: These essays are provided for educational purposes only and do not constitute medical advice from the author. They are meant to be concise and digestible, and they should not be considered comprehensive. The information in the books and web sites to which this manuscript links should also not be used as the basis for diagnosing or treating any medical condition. Some of the material presented is based upon the author's personal experience and not drawn from formally published studies. Some explanations regarding the causes of disease are not scientifically precise because they are meant to convey general ideas to patients. In addition, many treatments discussed are not FDA-approved and are mentioned for use in an off-label manner. The author does not have an endorsement agreement with any of the drugs mentioned. Specific brand names are mentioned solely for the sake of providing readers with examples they will recognize when filling prescriptions or purchasing over-the-counter medications. Generic names for many pharmaceuticals are listed in parentheses immediately after brand names. Since publication, important information may have been published that contradicts information provided within this book. Any decisions you make in regard to your health or your patients' health should be made with the counsel of a board-certified dermatologist.

Acknowledgments

My many teachers and professors at Randolph High School, the University of Michigan, the University of Virginia, Motefiore Medical Center, the University of Medicine and Dentistry of New Jersey, and the Roswell Park Cancer Institute were particularly instrumental in my development as a student and professional. Without all their support, I would not have had the opportunity to practice dermatology.

I am also grateful for my parents, the entire staff at Randolph Dermatology and Mohs Micrographic Surgery, Randolph Medical and Renal Associates, and all the local physicians around Randolph, New Jersey, for helping support my practice.

I sincerely thank my patients for their cooperation and inspiring enthusiasm in helping make this book a reality.

Most of all, I would like to thank my wife, Lauren, and son, Alex, for their unconditional love and support.

Identifying Your Skin Condition

Want to find out what your skin condition might be called? Use the table below to see how the most common skin conditions present. The term *present* is used throughout this book and, in a medical context, means the way in which a skin condition first appears to the patient. As always, consult with your dermatologist to learn exactly what you have—this table is just a starting point.

What You Observe	What the Condition Might Be
Acne	Acne
	Folliculitis
	Pseudofolliculitis Barbae
	Rosacea
Acne-like spots on the arms	Keratosis Pilaris
Acne-like spots on the body	Acne
	Folliculitis
	Grover's Disease
Painful reddish bumps (boils) in the groin or armpits	Abscess
	Cyst
	Hidradenitis Suppurativa
Painful reddish bumps (boils) on the face	Abscess
	Acne
	Cyst
	Rosacea
Painful reddish bumps (boils) elsewhere	Abscess
	Cyst

What You Observe	**What the Condition Might Be**
Itchy dry skin	Dry Skin
	Eczema
	Psoriasis
	Seborrheic Dermatitis
Itchy open wounds—can't stop picking them	Prurigo Nodularis
Itchy, pink, flaky patches	Allergic Contact Dermatitis
	Candidiasis
	Cheilitis
	Dermatophyte Infection
	Eczema
	Erythrasma
	Intertrigo
	Lupus
	Pityriasis Rosea
	Psoriasis
	Scabies
	Seborrheic Dermatitis
	Stasis Dermatitis
Itchy, pink, non-flaky patches—come and go quickly	Hives
Itchy, pink, non-flaky patches—after sun exposure	Polymorphous Light Eruption
Itchy pink or brown leathery patches	Lichen Simplex Chronicus
Itchy purple bumps	Lichen Planus
Itchy skin on mid-back—may look normal or dark brown	Macular Amyloidosis
	Notalgia Paresthetica
Non-itchy pink patches	Basal Cell Carcinoma
	Erythrasma
	Granuloma Fissuratum
	Lupus
	Mycosis Fungoides
	Pityriasis Rosea
	Poikiloderma
	Porokeratosis
	Psoriasis
	Seborrheic Dermatitis
	Squamous Cell Carcinoma
Non-itchy red or purple spots and patches	Cherry Angioma
	Leukocytoclastic Vasculitis
	Pigmented Purpura
Non-itchy whitish patches	Pityriasis Alba
	Tinea Versicolor
	Vitiligo

The Skinny on Skin

What You Observe	**What the Condition Might Be**
Black spots, patches, or bumps	Melanoma
Brown or tan spots or bumps	Dermatofibroma
	Dysplastic Mole
	Lentigo
	Melasma
	Mole
	Seborrheic Keratosis
	Skin Tag
	Wart
Fluid or pus-filled bumps	Acne
	Bullous Pemphigoid
	Folliculitis
	Herpes
	Hidradenitis Suppurativa
	Pemphigus
	Rosacea
	Shingles
Lump under the skin	Acne
	Cyst
	Erythema Nodosum
	Hidradenitis Suppurativa
	Lipoma
	Rosacea
Pink spots or bumps	Actinic Keratosis
	Angiofibroma
	Basal Cell Carcinoma
	Cherry Angioma
	Chondrodermatitis Nodularis Helicis
	Dermatofibroma
	Granuloma Annulare
	Granuloma Fissuratum
	Mole
	Molluscum Contagiosum
	Squamous Cell Carcinoma
Tender, firm, reddish skin on the lower legs	Lipodermatosclerosis
Tender reddish lumps on the lower legs	Erythema Nodosum
Tiny tan or pinkish bumps with a dimple on the face	Sebaceous Hyperplasia
Whitish spots on the lips	Fordyce Granules

What You Observe	What the Condition Might Be
Crumbling thin nails	Lichen Planus
Nails separating from the nail bed	Onycholysis
Rash around nails	Paronychia
Yellow nails	Dermatophyte Infection
	Psoriasis
Excess sweating	Hyperhidrosis
Hair loss	Alopecia Areata
	Androgenetic Alopecia
	Dermatophyte Infection
	Lichen Planus
	Lupus
	Telogen Effluvium
Painful open wounds	Hidradenitis Suppurativa
	Pyoderma Gangrenosum
Sores in the mouth	Aphthous Ulcer
	Lichen Planus
	Lupus
	Pemphigus

The Skinny on Skin

Part I
Medical Skin Conditions

Acne

Acne is probably the most common condition for which patients visit dermatologists. What appears to be a mild case can actually have a major psychological impact on the patient. Acne presents with whiteheads, blackheads, pink bumps, pus-filled bumps, and painful lumps under the skin. Treatment involves the use of cleansers, creams, or oral antibiotics. While these treatments suppress acne, the condition tends to recur if treatment is stopped. Fortunately, acne may resolve by the mid- to late twenties.

Most treatments take a few weeks to start working, peak in efficacy after two months, and provide about 30 percent improvement. Expect slow, incremental improvement—not rapid, overnight clearance. For example, someone presenting with one hundred acne lesions can expect to see about seventy lesions two months after beginning a single treatment. After two months, when the medicines are fully working, return to the office so the dermatologist can adjust the treatment routine if needed.

SKIN CLEANSING

Gentle skin cleansers are recommended for all acne patients. A favored prescription strength cleanser is a 10% sulfacetamide wash with or without 5% sulfur, which is applied to the face for two minutes, then rinsed off. Use the wash in the morning, after showering, and again at bedtime. Weaker medicated cleansers are available without a prescription.

RETINOIDS

Retinoid creams, including Differin (adapalene), Retin-A (tretinoin), and Tazorac (tazarotene) are the first-line acne treatments. Apply one of these creams at night after washing your face with a cleanser, as described above. Begin by applying a small pea-sized drop of cream to the tip of an index finger, and then rub that cream into all the fingers. Finally, spread the cream onto the entire face, avoiding your upper and lower eyelids.

Retinoid creams are not designed to work by spot treating, and they are not designed to work by applying them only when breakouts are occurring. Instead, apply the cream to the entire face on a regular basis to reduce the frequency and severity of breakouts over the long term. Applying too much cream too fast, however, can cause skin dryness, peeling, redness, and itching. Therefore, start by applying a small amount of cream every other night. If the cream is tolerated, after two weeks try using it every night.

If dryness and peeling ensue, try applying a smaller amount. Placing a product like Cetaphil facial moisturizer right over the retinoid cream at night and throughout the day will also reduce dryness and peeling. Finally, cutting back the frequency of application will reduce irritation. These creams may still work if used only every third or fourth night.

Retinoid creams work by cleaning out the pores that cause acne. A few weeks after starting treatment, some patients notice their acne looks worse. The medicine is unclogging the pores, and the contents of the pores come up to the skin surface where you can see them. Hang in there! Within a few weeks, things will settle down as the pores clear out, and continued improvement will follow. Two months after starting treatment, patients can expect about 30 percent improvement. Finally, in the summer, consider wearing a hat or applying sunscreen during the day, because retinoid creams can make your skin sensitive to the sun.

OTHER TREATMENTS

A sulfacetamide cleanser and retinoid cream are not sufficient to clear many patients' skin. Other treatments commonly needed in these cases include Finacea (azeleic acid gel), Aczone (dapsone gel), and sulfacetamide creams or lotions with or without 5% sulfur. These products need a few weeks of use to start working, and they do not fully kick in until two months, after which time you can expect about 30 percent improvement from any one treatment.

As with the retinoid creams discussed above, these medications are not designed to work by spot treating, and they are not designed to work by applying them only when breakouts are occurring. Instead, patients need to use them on a regular basis to reduce the frequency and severity of breakouts over the long term. Apply a very thin layer to the entire face after washing with a cleanser in the morning or evening, as described above.

More severe acne or acne that presents with painful lumps un-

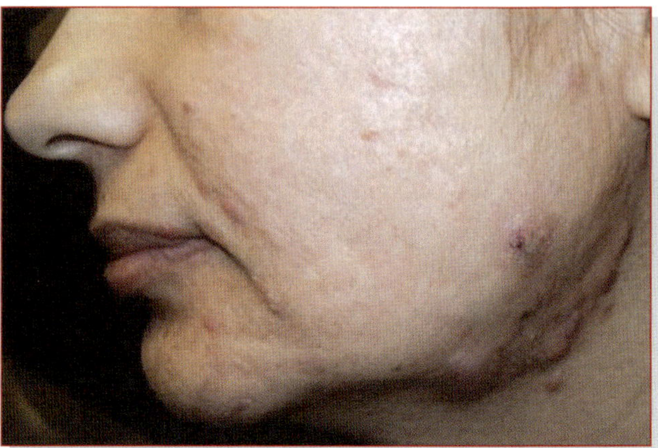

Cystic acne

derneath the skin may require oral antibiotics. Read more about this treatment option in Part II of this book. Women may also consider using oral contraceptives for acne not responding to conventional creams. Severe acne that does not respond to standard creams, washes, oral antibiotics, or oral contraceptives may respond to Accutane (isotretinoin), which is the only treatment that sometimes leads to a permanent cure. See Part II of this book for a description of this medication.

Actinic Keratosis

The phrase *actinic keratosis* (ak-tin´ik ker-ă-tō´sis) means "growth from too much sunlight." Actinic keratoses are pink rough spots, most commonly found on the face, ears, scalp, back of the hands, and forearms. They occur most frequently in sun worshippers. Actinic keratoses are often referred to as precancerous because a small percentage of them develop into a squamous cell carcinoma after a few years.

Dermatologists treat actinic keratoses by spraying them with ice-cold liquid nitrogen, which causes a localized frostbite in the area. The lesions scab up and peel off within a week or so. Immediately after treatment, the site can look like an insect bite— so if you have an important social engagement within the next week, treatment can be deferred until a later date. No special skin care is needed after treatments.

The frostbite created by liquid nitrogen could cause a fluid-filled blister to form in the area. These freeze blisters heal up within a few days without any treatment. There is also a small chance that a second freeze will be required to get rid of the actinic keratosis. Therefore, if a keratosis is still there one month after treatment, return for a touch-up session. Finally, treated skin can develop a light-colored tone.

Some patients have so many actinic keratoses that it is impractical to treat them with liquid nitrogen because it would hurt too much. These patients may benefit from Aldara (imiquimod cream) or Efudex (5 fluorouracil cream). Use gloves when handling these creams, and don't apply them in or around the eyes. Apply a thin layer of Aldara cream to the affected field of skin at nighttime, after washing, on Monday, Wednesday, and Friday, for about twelve weeks. Wash off the cream the morning after application. When using Efudex, apply a thin layer of cream to the affected field of skin, after washing, both in the morning and the evening for three weeks.

Skin treated with Aldara or Efudex looks red and crusty. Most patients are surprised at just how red and crusty the skin can look. Patients considering using these creams should find images of skin treated with Aldara or Efudex so they know what to expect. It is not a good idea to use these creams if you have important social engagements on the calendar during the treatment phase or up to one month after treatment.

Once you initiate therapy, apply a moisturizer, such as Cetaphil, in the morning and throughout the day to treat any scabs that form. Moreover, stop the cream and consult your doctor if you develop discomfort at the treatment site.

Some patients with many actinic keratoses cannot tolerate having a reddish face for many weeks at a time. They may benefit from chemical peels, which can remove actinic keratoses in one or two sessions. Each session leaves the face pink for a few days, and the skin may peel for a week or two afterward. Fridays are a good time to perform chemical peels, because it gives the patient the weekend to recover. See Part III of this book for more information about chemical peels.

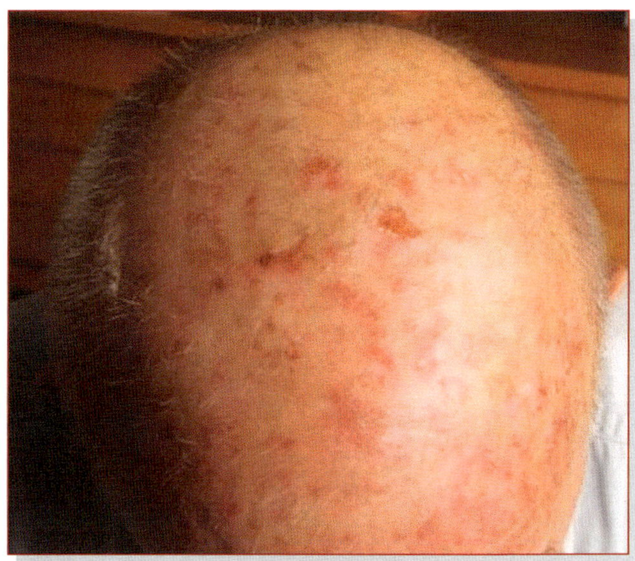

Actinic keratoses

Finally, patients with actinic keratoses are at risk for skin cancer and should consider getting a full skin examination to rule out this possibility. Reducing sun exposure may also pare the odds of developing additional actinic keratoses in the decades ahead. For advice on sun protection, see the beginning of the essay "Skin Aging: Prevention and Treatment" in Part I of this book.

Allergic Contact Dermatitis

Allergic contact dermatitis presents as an itchy, pink rash. This condition develops when a chemical or material touches the skin and tricks the immune system into thinking an infectious agent has landed on the skin. The immune system then mistakenly sends T cells to the skin to fight an infection that does not exist. Once in the skin, the T cells release chemicals that cause the redness and itching. Sometimes the rash arises on only a certain area of the body, but it may present all over the body.

Allergic contact dermatitis can result from exposure to any of thousands of chemicals or materials. Common causes of this condition include perfumes, the oil in poison ivy leaves, nickel in jewelry, antibiotic creams, hair dyes, preservatives in shampoos, and adhesives used for press-on nails, but the list of all possible causes is endless. Some patients develop the rash after the first chemical or material exposure, but others can develop a rash after years of exposure without incident.

Once the rash starts, it usually lasts around three weeks and then disappears, providing one is no longer exposed to the chemical. This means that a chemical can cause a persistent rash even if the chemical is only touching the skin once every three weeks or so. It also means that patients may need at least three weeks of treatment. If one treats the skin for two weeks and then stops, the rash may come back.

The first-line therapy is a corticosteroid cream, such as hydrocortisone, triamcinalone, synalar, or clobetasol. These creams work by removing T cells from the skin and function best if applied immediately after bathing, when the skin is still damp. Apply the cream later in the day if needed—particularly before bedtime to avoid nighttime itching. Typically, allergic contact dermatitis will resolve after several days, when you can stop the cream and apply a bland moisturizer, such as Vaseline or Cetaphil. If the dermatitis recurs, reapply the corticosteroid cream daily until improvement is seen.

Corticosteroid creams applied on a daily basis for weeks to months with no breaks can slowly start to thin out the skin. In this case, it could look shiny and wrinkled, and tiny blood vessels could appear in the skin. For this reason, if you have used the cream daily for two weeks in a row, take a two-week break or switch to weekend use only for a while before restarting it. Moisturize your skin during the break in therapy.

A real cure, not just relief, is attainable by identifying the offending chemical or material and keeping it away from the skin. A patch test is advisable to find the guilty chemical, because patients and dermatologists cannot routinely specify the allergen without it. Patch testing is described in Part IV of this book. If the test reveals a true allergy, you will be given a list of skin and hair care products that will be safe to use.

If you lack access to patch testing, consider stopping the use of perfumes, nail treatments, antibiotic creams, and jewelry. Also consider using hypoallergenic and fragrance free skin and hair care products, soaps, antiperspirants, and detergents.

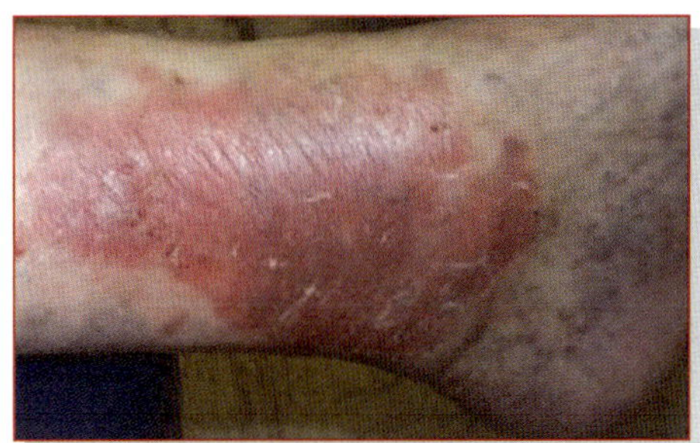

Dermatitis of the left leg. After a patch test revealed a skin allergy to Neosporin, the patient remembered recently using Neosporin to treat leg itch.

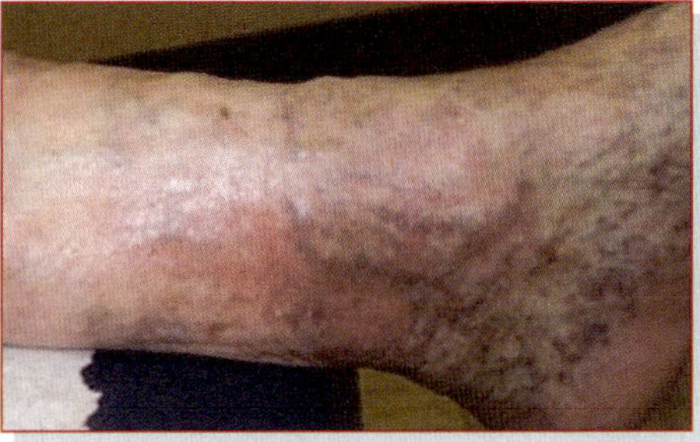

Clearance of dermatitis with clobetasol cream.

Part I Medical Skin Conditions

Alopecia Areata (Hair Loss)

Alopecia areata (al-ō-pē´shē-ă area´ta) usually appears as oval-shaped areas of hair loss on the scalp or beard area. Uncommonly, alopecia areata can lead to hair loss over the entire scalp or, even less commonly, the entire body.

Alopecia areata is considered an autoimmune condition caused when the immune system mistakenly sends T cells to the skin to fight an infection that does not exist. The immune cells cause inflammation in the area, leading to hair loss. The condition probably results from the combination of genes inherited from one's parents, since the genes are what largely program the immune system how to respond to different stimuli. Patients sometimes develop other genetically related autoimmune diseases, including

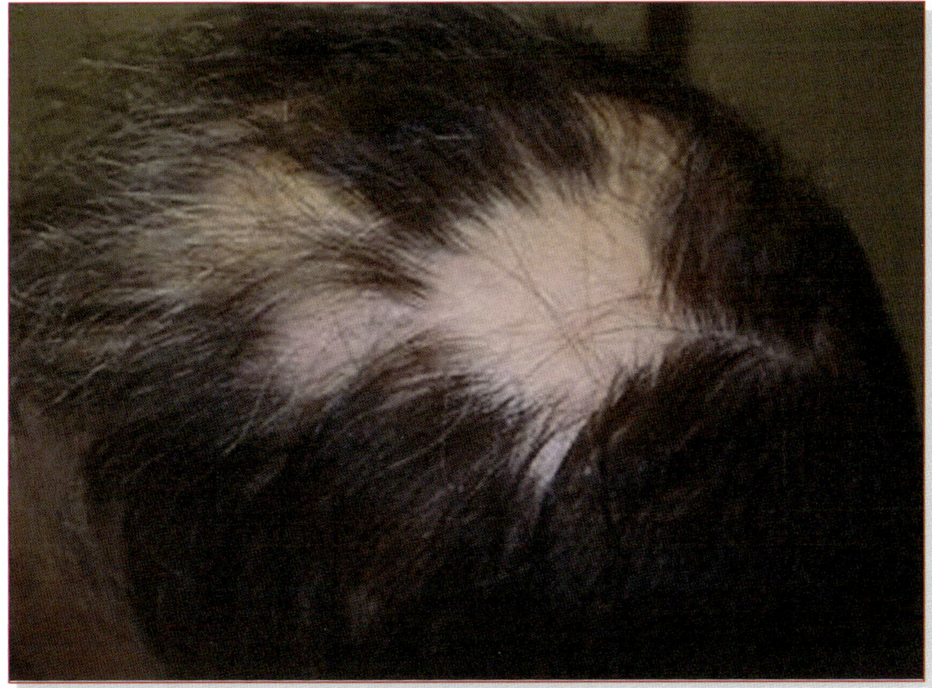

Alopecia areata

---

eczema, vitiligo, diabetes, inflammatory bowel disease, and thyroid disease. Those demonstrating obvious signs of these conditions may be tested for them.

The natural course of alopecia areata is different in every patient. For example, patches of hair loss may resolve on their own with no treatment. On the other hand, patches could last for years if untreated. Patches could enlarge or stay the same size—it is impossible to predict what will happen for any given patient.

The treatment of choice consists of monthly injections into the area of hair loss with a corticosteroid called triamcinalone. Triamcinalone suppresses the immune system in the skin for weeks, allowing hair to grow back. Several treatments are usually required before hair regrowth is noticed.

If hair loss involves more than a small area, treatment with a sensitizing chemical, such as diphenylcyclopropenone or Anthralin (dithranol), may be an appropriate option. The medication is formulated as a liquid (diphenylcyclopropenone) or cream (Anthralin) and applied to the scalp on a periodic basis until a mild rash develops, and after many months, irritation from the rash stimulates hair growth. Finally, if hair loss affects the entire scalp or the entire body, immunosuppressive medications may help achieve hair regrowth. Unfortunately, when the pills are stopped hair loss may recur.

Androgenetic Alopecia (Hair Loss)

Androgenetic alopecia (an-drō-jen´et-ik al-ō-pē´shē-ǎ) may occur in men or women. This type of hair loss results from inheriting a certain combination of genes from one's parents. Patients may have one or more relatives with hair loss, including siblings, parents, grandparents, aunts, uncles, or cousins. Other patients may report no family history of hair loss.

Androgenetic alopecia presents as a slowly progressive decline in scalp-hair density. The scalp becomes more and more visible with time. In fact, hairs are shrinking in size. Patients do not typically report excessive hair shedding in the sink or on the brush. In men, hair loss usually occurs in a typical pattern: male pattern hair loss. In women, hair loss may begin with the forehead and extend back to the top of the scalp.

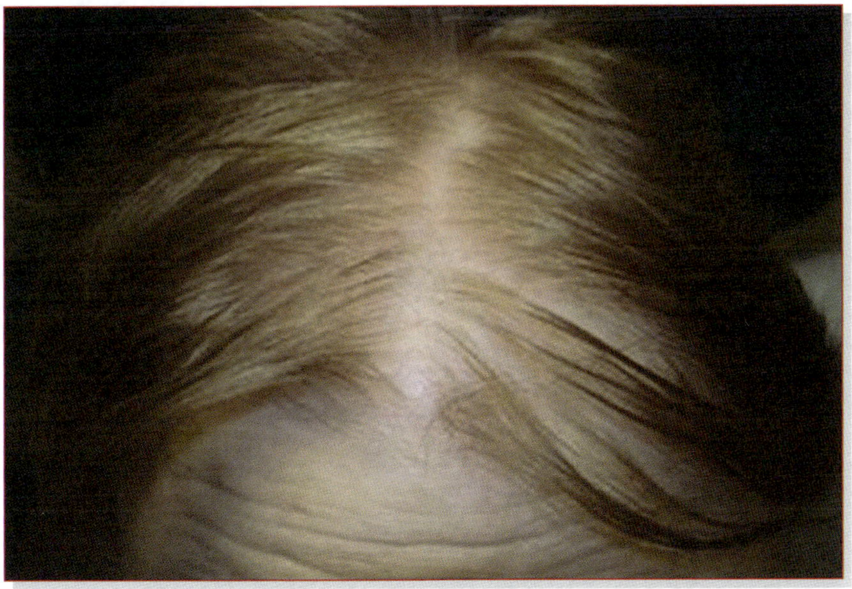

Androgenetic alopecia in a woman

Minoxidil, the active ingredient in Rogaine, is a first-line treatment for androgenetic alopecia. It is available without a prescription. Minoxidil is applied twice a day, and it may take a few months to see results. This medicine is available in solution and foam formulations, and it comes in 2 and 5 percent concentrations. The foam absorbs better into the scalp, while the solution may drip down onto the cheeks, where it could grow hair. Patients who attain good results with minoxidil should discontinue it with some caution, because one may gradually lose the progress one had earned.

For men, Propecia (finasteride) is also available. This pill is taken daily, and results are seen after a few months. A very small percentage of men on the drug develop lowered sex drive, which is typically reversible once the medicine is discontinued. Like Rogaine, if Propecia is stopped for long enough, one may gradually lose the progress one had attained. Unfortunately, Propecia does not work for women. Finally, many pregnant women report enhanced hair growth while on prenatal vitamins, so this intervention may be worth a try.

Angiofibroma

Angiofibromas (an´jē-ō-fī-brō´măs) are harmless pink or skin-colored bumps that typically arise on or around the nose. Doctors haven't concluded why they form. Since angiofibromas are harmless, they require no treatment when they appear in isolation. Patients who present with clusters of angiofibromas, however, need further evaluation for a condition called tuberous sclerosis.

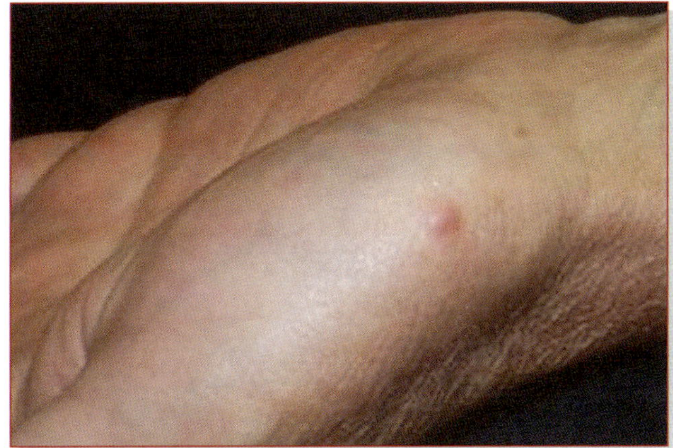
Angiofibroma

Aphthous Ulcer

Aphthous (af´thŭs) ulcers, also called canker sores, are painful wounds that form in the mouth. They usually resolve without treatment in a week or two, but they may recur—sometimes for years. Recurrent aphthous ulcers are common, affecting up to 25 percent of the population.

It is difficult to find the cause of aphthous ulcers, and in some cases the cause is never found. In other patients, however, the condition may be triggered by oral trauma, the cessation of smoking, anxiety or stress, hormonal changes related to the menstrual cycle, or sensitivity to food ingredients, such as benzoic acid or cinnamaldehyde. A patch test is available to detect allergies to benzoic acid and cinnamaldehyde. See Part II of this book for more information about this test. Ulcerations may also result from deficiencies in iron, vitamin B12, and folate, and blood tests can evaluate this possibility.

Certain systemic diseases can also present with aphthous ulcers. Examples of such conditions include Behcet's syndrome, gluten-sensitive bowel disease, inflammatory bowel disease, and HIV. Patients who have symptoms of these conditions may be tested for them.

Pharmaceuticals such as nonsteroidal anti-inflammatory medicines (aspirin, ibuprofen, and naprosyn) and beta-blockers (metoprolol) have also been associated with the development of aphthous ulcers. Tell your doctor if you started taking any new medicines around the time of ulcer formation.

Cytomegalovirus and the herpes virus can cause outbreaks resembling aphthous ulcers. Herpes outbreaks tend to occur in the exact same location with every recurrence—often on the tongue or palate. A viral culture can determine if the ulcers are caused by herpes or cytomegalovirus. Read the chapter titled "Herpes" in Part I of this book for more information on the subject.

The goal of treatment is to reduce the pain and duration of breakouts. Avoid oral trauma from hard toothbrushes and acidic food and drinks. The first-line therapy is a corticosteroid, such as triamcinalone, formulated as a dental paste. Apply this paste to ulcers up to five times a day until ulcers heal. The use of Listerine mouthwash twice a day may also reduce the pain and duration of ulcers. Another anti-inflammatory product, 5 percent Amlexanox paste (Aphthasol or Aptheal), applied to ulcers two to four times daily may reduce the size, pain, and duration of ulcers. If topical treatments fail, a short course of prednisone may be considered. Finally, after the condition resolves, using mouthwashes containing triclosan, such as Plax and Total, twice a day may reduce the likelihood of ulcer recurrences.

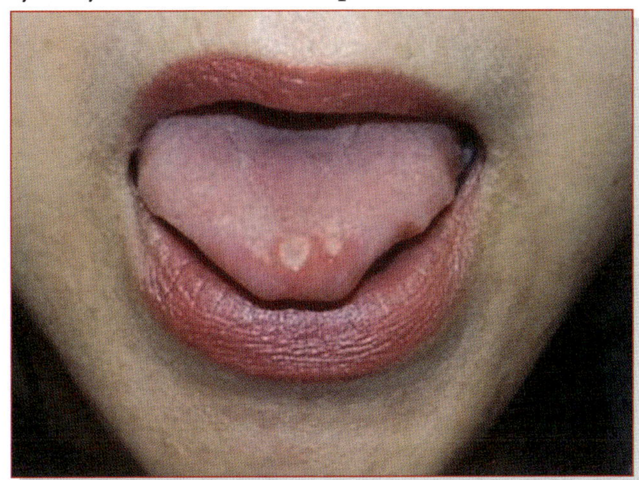

Aphthous ulcers

Basal Cell Carcinoma

Basal cell carcinoma (bā´săl sel kar-si-nō´mă) is the most common type of cancer that arises in the population. It results from the damaging effects of sun exposure over a period of decades. The growth typically appears as a flat pink patch or as a raised, shiny bump that enlarges by a few millimeters every year. The surface may have a scab and bleed with minor trauma. Basal cell carcinomas almost never spread to other parts of the body.

Thankfully, there are many excellent treatments for basal cell carcinoma that do not require chemotherapy and radiation. Moreover, as long as you seek treatment in a timely manner, it should not alter your life span. If the cancer is below the neck and has not spread deeply into the skin, the dermatologist may treat it with a cream called Aldara (imiquimod). At night the patient applies the cream to the growth, and a small area of normal-looking skin around it, and rinses it off in the morning. Applications are repeated five nights per week, usually Monday through Friday, for approximately six weeks. The area becomes very red and crusty during treatment, and patients should consider the cosmetic effects before proceeding with this technique. Stop the cream and consult your doctor if you develop discomfort at the treatment site. In addition, Efudex (5-fluorouracil cream) applied twice daily for up to six weeks works in a manner similar to Aldara.

The dermatologist may also treat superficial carcinomas with electrodessication and curettage. With this technique, the doctor injects the growth with lidocaine to numb the area. An instrument then makes the cancer form a scab, which is scraped away painlessly. This procedure takes about fifteen minutes.

A third method of treating superficial basal cell carcinomas uses liquid nitrogen, which the dermatologist sprays onto the spot, causing a localized frostbite reaction. The skin cancer forms a scab within about two weeks and then falls off. This procedure takes approximately one minute. The disadvantage of liquid nitrogen,

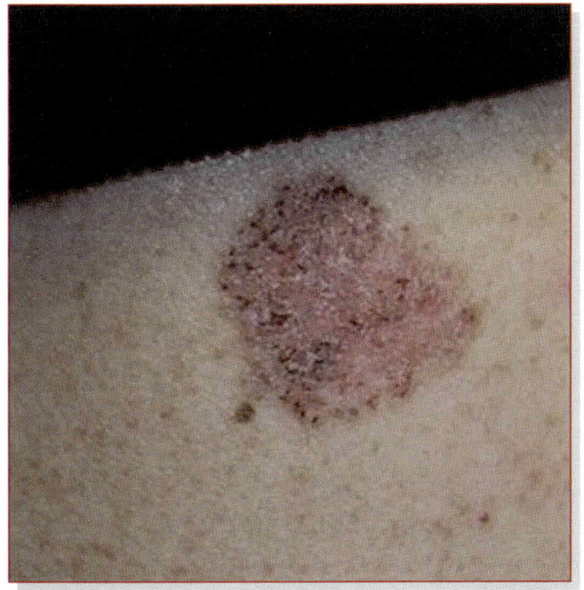

Basal cell carcinoma presenting as a flat pink patch on the left back

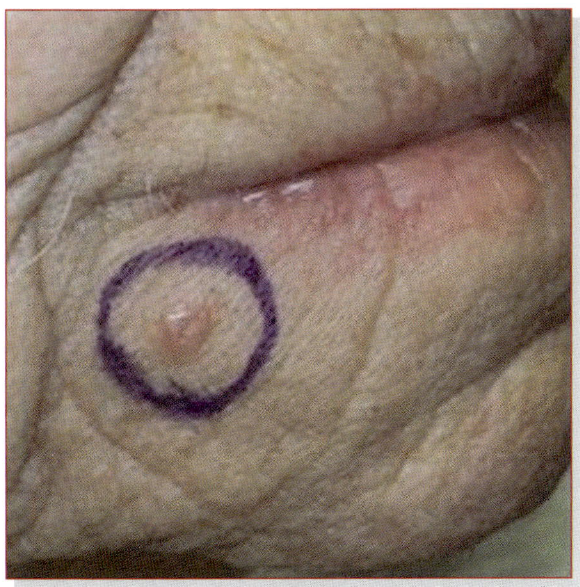

Basal cell carcinoma presenting as a raised shiny growth

electrodessication and curettage, and Aldara and Efudex creams is that patients never receive confirmation from a pathologist that the cancer is all out.

If the cancer is not superficial and has spread deeply into the skin, the dermatologist may need to excise the growth. He or she first injects lidocaine around the lesion to numb the area. The doctor then removes more tissue around the spot in a painless manner with a scalpel. Finally, sutures are placed to close the surgical site and will need to be removed in about two weeks. The entire process requires one hour. Afterward, the specimen is submitted to a pathologist to confirm it was completely removed. Excisions are also reasonable for superficial basal cell carcinomas because they confirm the cancer is completely out. Read more about excisions in Part IV of this book.

Finally, if the skin cancer is very large, on the face, or is recurrent, Mohs micrographic surgery should be considered. Mohs surgeons are dermatologists with special training who perform this procedure in the office. The surgeon first injects lidocaine around the growth to numb the area. He or she then removes the cancer and a small moat of normal looking skin around it with a scalpel. The same doctor then examines the specimen under the microscope while you wait in the office to confirm that it has been removed completely. Once it's all out, the surgeon repairs the site. This method is discussed in greater detail in Part IV of this book.

Patients with basal cell carcinoma could develop a second skin cancer and need a full skin examination to make sure the rest of the skin is normal. It is also important for patients to limit their sun exposure to help prevent the development of additional skin cancers in the decades ahead. For advice on sun protection, see the beginning of the essay "Skin Aging: Prevention and Treatment" in Part I of this book.

Candidiasis

Candidiasis (kan-di-dīă-sis) is a skin infection caused by the yeast *Candida*. It presents as itchy, reddish patches of skin with reddish bumps surrounding the patches. *Candida* prefers to live on warm, moist surfaces. Therefore, it usually arises in the groin area or under the breasts. Occasionally, candidiasis presents in other skin folds—such as between the fingers and in the skin folds around the fingernails. It may also arise on the warm, moist backs of bedridden patients. In this case, it may appear as scattered, pus-filled bumps.

Candidiasis responds to creams, such as nystatin cream or ketoconazole cream. Patients should apply the prescribed cream twice daily for about a month, but obese and diabetic patients may require longer treatment times to clear the rash. Once the skin clears, stop the creams and apply nystatin or miconazole powder after bathing to prevent recurrences. Desenex and Zeasorb are brands of antifungal powders available without a prescription. Weight loss in obese patients and better glucose control in diabetic patients may reduce the risk of recurrence.

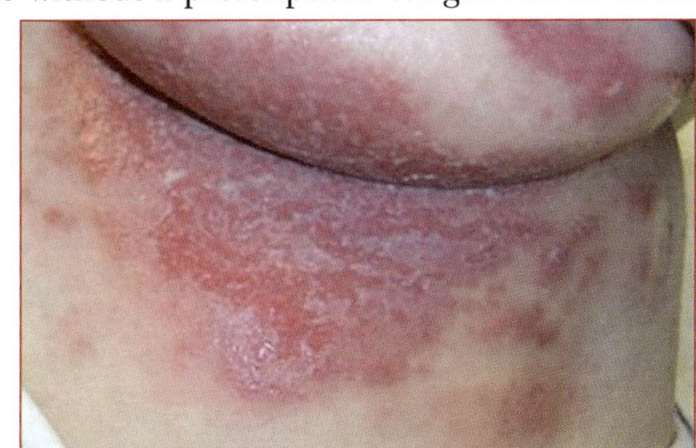

Candidiasis of the left chest

Cheilitis

Cheilitis (kī-lī´tis) presents as flaky, pink skin along the border of the lips. There are a number of possible causes. For example, angular cheilitis, which presents at the corners of the lips, is typically caused by overgrowth of *Candida* yeast. Angular cheilitis responds well to nystatin cream applied three times daily. Sometimes drooling during sleep can aggravate this condition. Applying a barrier cream, like Desitin, to affected areas at bedtime may protect skin from saliva. Desitin cream is available without a prescription.

Cheilitis may also present all around the lips. This type of cheilitis may result from a skin allergy to chemicals in lipstick, lip gloss, toothpaste, or mouthwash. In this case, a patch test may help reveal the guilty chemical. The patch test is described in detail in Part IV of this book.

If patch testing does not reveal the cause of the cheilitis, other possibilities should be considered. For example, irritant contact dermatitis is another cause of cheilitis all around the lips. This condition results from exposure to an irritating chemical. This is not an allergic reaction but an irritant reaction. Lip licking, lipstick, and consumption of some medications are possible causes of irritant contact dermatitis on the lips. Stopping exposure to the irritating chemical cures irritant contact dermatitis.

Endogenous cheilitis is another cause of cheilitis all around the lips. Endogenous cheilitis is an autoimmune condition, caused when the immune system mistakenly sends plasma cells to the lips to fight an infection that does not exist. A biopsy may be needed to confirm the diagnosis. Corticosteroid creams, such as hydrocortisone, and nonsteroidal anti-inflammatory creams, such as Elidel (pimecrolimus cream), treat this condition. Unfortunately, when the creams are stopped, the condition may recur.

In even rarer circumstances, vitamin deficiency can cause cheilitis around the mouth. If this is suspected, blood tests can rule out vitamin B12 and iron deficiencies.

A condition called contact urticaria can resemble cheilitis. Contact urticaria presents as itching, stinging, tingling, or swelling after eating certain foods. Foods commonly causing contact urticaria include apples, mangos, oranges, tomatoes, and kiwis. Keeping a food diary may reveal if foods are causing the problem.

Less common causes of cheilitis include cheilitis glandularis and granulomatous cheilitis. A skin biopsy is required to diagnose these conditions.

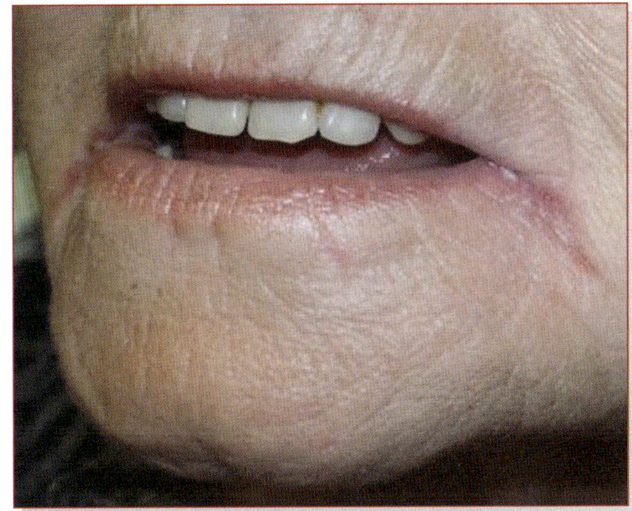

Angular cheilitis

Cherry Angioma

Cherry angiomas (an-jē-ō´măs) are harmless, tiny, cherry-colored spots or bumps. Under a microscope, they appear as dilated and twisted blood vessels, but doctors don't know why they arise. Angiomas are extremely common—almost all adults have at least a few of them. Most times they stay rather tiny, but in some cases they can enlarge. Dermatologists treat cherry angiomas with a technique called electrodessication. The dermatologist may first inject the growth with lidocaine to numb the area. An instrument then makes the angioma form a scab, which peels off in a week or two. If a month has gone by and the spot is not completely gone, return to the office for a touch-up session.

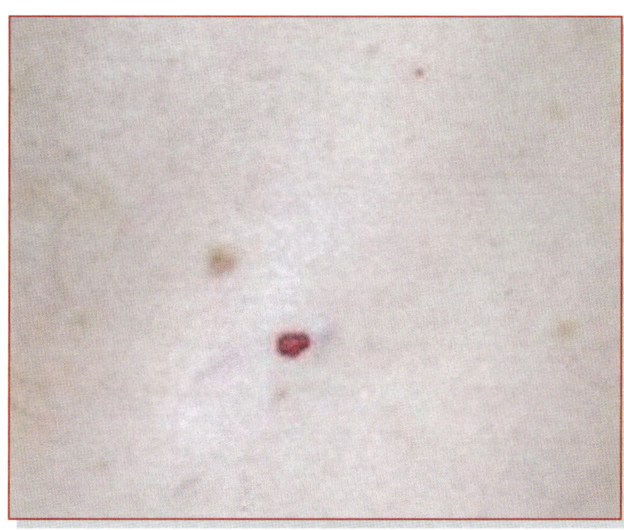

Cherry angioma

Chondrodermatitis Nodularis Helicis

Chondrodermatitis nodularis helicis (kon-drō-der-ma-tī´tis nod-yū-lar´is hel´i-sis) presents as a painful bump on the top of the ear. It arises from too much pressure on the ear that ensues from sleeping on the same side over a long period of time. Dermatologists cannot always easily differentiate chondrodermatitis from skin cancer. For this reason, a skin biopsy may be necessary to confirm the diagnosis.

Changing your sleep position helps resolve the condition by reducing pressure on the affected ear. You could also use a doughnut pillow with a hole in the middle to relieve pressure on the ear during sleep. Doughnut pillows may be found at surgical supply stores. Other treatments include corticosteroid creams and corticosteroid injections.

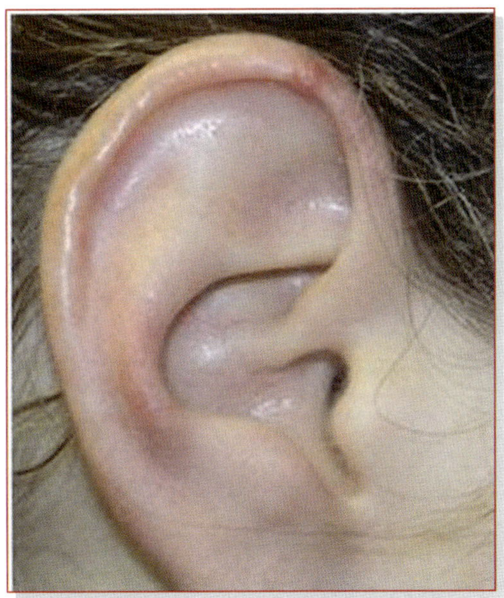

Chondrodermatitis nodularis helicis

Cyst

Cysts are noncancerous growths that present under the skin. They are typically firm, smooth, and round. A cyst is really a sack filled with a malodorous white or black material called keratin. Sometimes there is a tunnel that connects the cyst to the surface of the skin. Doctors don't know for sure why cysts form.

A cyst typically just sits there and causes no problems. However, the sack can break, sometimes from physical trauma. When this happens, the keratin leaks out into the surrounding skin. Your immune system mistakes this keratin for an infectious agent, resulting in a great deal of inflammation. Redness, swelling, and discomfort can arise, and the keratin can drain onto the surface of the skin through the cyst's tunnel. The whole scenario resembles a volcanic eruption. Injecting a corticosteroid such as triamcinalone into the area helps calm down inflammation.

If the cyst is causing no problems, it does not need treatment. However, removing a cyst may preempt a painful eruption. To remove the cyst, the dermatologist injects the growth with lidocaine to numb the area. Then, he or she creates a small opening above the cyst with a scalpel and squeezes the cyst out of the opening. Sutures are used to close the opening. Patients should schedule a forty-five-minute appointment for this procedure and usually return in two weeks for suture removal.

A very tiny type of cyst called a milium also commonly arises in adult facial skin. Milia look like tiny whiteheads. Fortunately, they do not cause any problems, but they may persist for years. Dermatologists remove milia in the office with a needle by gently pricking the skin surface over the lesion. The dermatologist then uses a tiny metal instrument to push the milium out of the skin.

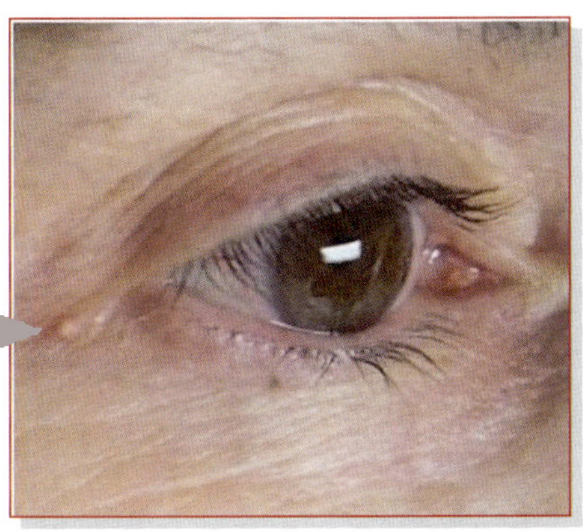

Milium

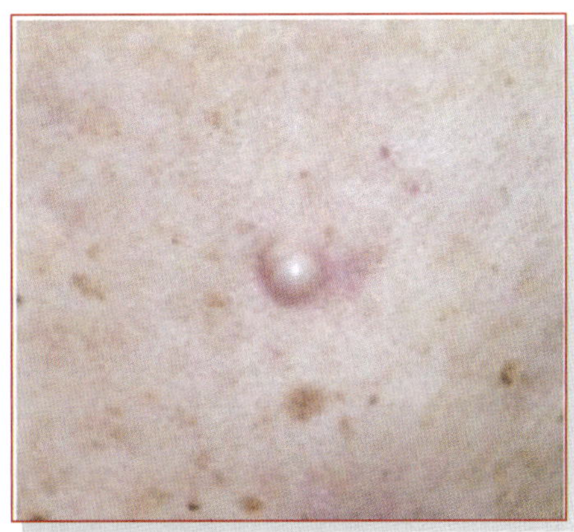

Cyst on the back

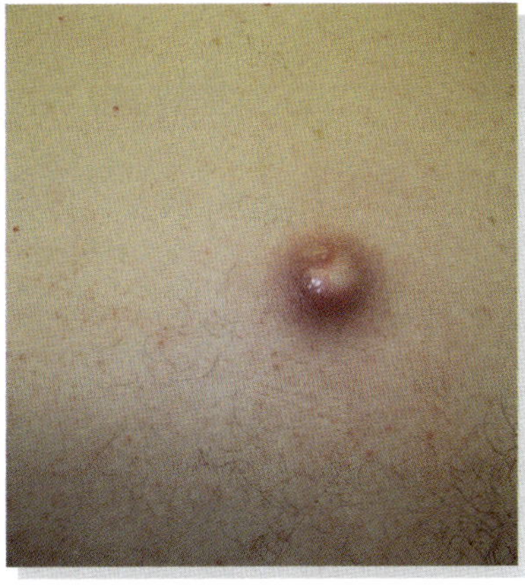

Inflamed cyst on the back

Highlights of a Cyst Excision

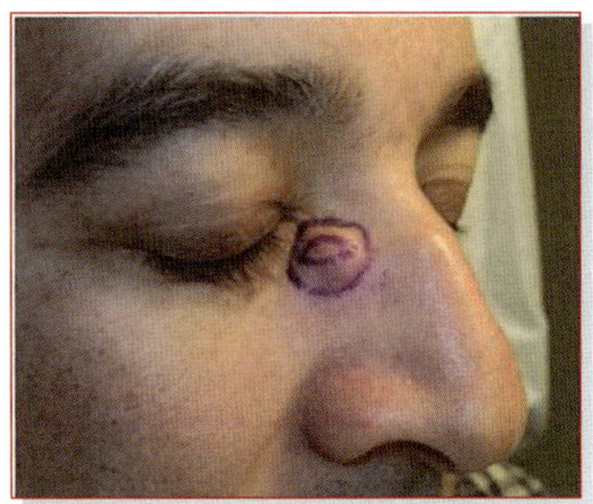

Cyst outlined with a
marking pen before removal

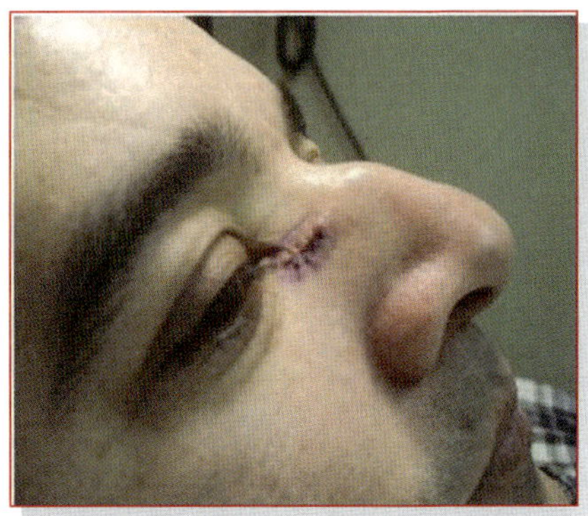

Sutures placed after cyst removed

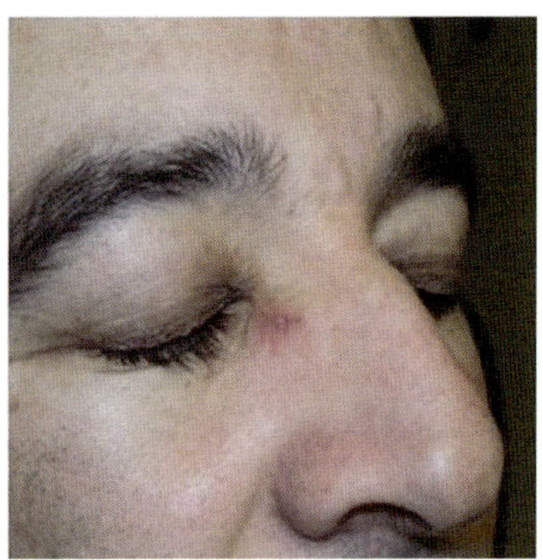

One week later, after suture removal

Part I Medical Skin Conditions

Dermatofibroma

Dermatofibromas (der´mă-tō-fi-brō´măs) are very common harmless skin growths that present as smooth, tan, brown, or pink firm bumps, usually about the size of a pencil eraser. The skin around them tends to form a dimple if squeezed. Dermatofibromas usually arise on the arms and legs and are less common elsewhere. The reason they form is unknown, but trauma to the skin from shaving or an insect bite may elicit them. Dermatofibromas may actually represent an abnormal healing response to trauma, but under a microscope a dermatofibroma looks different from a scar. A dermatofibroma is, therefore, similar to but not exactly a scar.

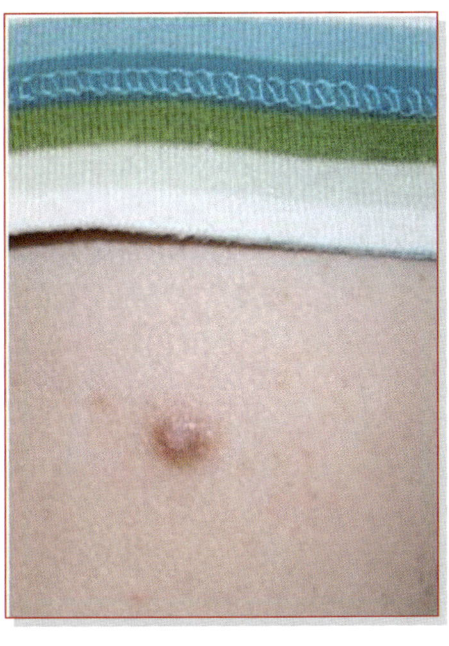

Dermatofibroma on the arm

Dermatofibromas usually stay the same size over time, but there is a small chance they may go away. They are not typically removed, however, because the risk of recurrence is high.

Dermatophyte Infection

Dermatophytes (der´mă-tō-fīts) are a type of fungus that causes some of the most common conditions for which patients present to dermatologists, including athlete's foot, jock itch, and ringworm. Dermatophytes may infect the hair, skin, or nails. These infections are easily passed from person to person by direct contact or by sharing brushes, towels, clothes, and shoes.

Antifungal creams are effective for treating most cases. Applying clotrimazole cream twice daily for four weeks eliminates most skin infections and is available over the counter without a prescription. Ketoconazole cream prescribed once or twice daily for approximately four weeks is an alternative. If the area is extensive, or if creams burn your skin, Lamisil (terbinafine) pills taken daily for two weeks work well.

Patients should avoid using corticosteroid creams on the rash while undergoing treatment. These creams are described in detail in Part II of this book. They may make the area less itchy, but these creams suppress the immune system in the local skin, making the fungal infection harder to cure. Treating itch with dermatophyte infections is difficult, because any anti-itch cream will provide moisture—which fungi thrive in. Scratching can irritate the skin further.

When dermatophytes infect the nails, they become yellow with a rough, crumbly appearance. However, yellow, rough-looking nails do not always indicate a fungal infection, because psoriasis of the nails can look the same. Therefore, before initiating treatment, the dermatologist should prove a fungal infection really exists by clipping a suspicious nail and sending it to a microbiologist to culture the organism and confirm its species. It takes about a month to get the result because dermatophytes grow very slowly. Once dermatophytes have infected the nails, they are very tough to get rid of. Cure rates for available medicines are not great, and recurrences are common.

Penlac (ciclopirox olamine) is the safest possible treatment of nail infections, but cure rates are low. Penlac is a nail lacquer that is painted onto affected nails daily. After a while a residue arises on the nail, and patients should scrape this off weekly with acetone and a file. Penlac can be used for up to forty-eight weeks. Another possible treatment is Lamisil (terbinafine). Patients must take Lamisil tablets for six weeks for fingernail infections and twelve weeks for toenail infections. Lamisil is generally safe and works better than Penlac, but in rare cases it causes serious side effects to the liver or a serious skin reaction. Patients considering Lamisil need a blood test to rule out preexisting liver disease. Once on therapy, patients should not drink alcohol. If side effects develop while you are on the medicine, stop taking it and call your doctor.

Dermatophyte infections of hair, called tinea capitis or ringworm, are common in children. Before initiating treatment, the dermatologist should prove a fungal infection really exists by sending some affected hairs to a microbiologist to culture the organism and confirm its species. When the diagnosis is strongly suspected or confirmed, the dermatologist should initiate treatment quickly, because infections can lead to permanent hair loss. Lamisil tablets are taken daily and not typically stopped until a few weeks after the infection visibly clears. Griseofulvin is an alternative medicine available in a liquid form. It is taken at twenty to twenty-five mg/kg/day for six to eight weeks and is typically not stopped until a few weeks after the infection visibly clears.

Importantly, dermatophytes thrive in moisture, so keeping the infected areas dry is crucial to clearing the infection and preventing it from coming back. Drying yourself thoroughly after showering or sweating is, therefore, essential. If the skin or toenails are or were infected, consider applying a powder to the affected area after showering or sweating. Do not apply antifungal cream at the same time, however, because the cream and powder will combine into a messy batter. Desenex and Zeasorb are brands of antifungal powders available without a prescription.

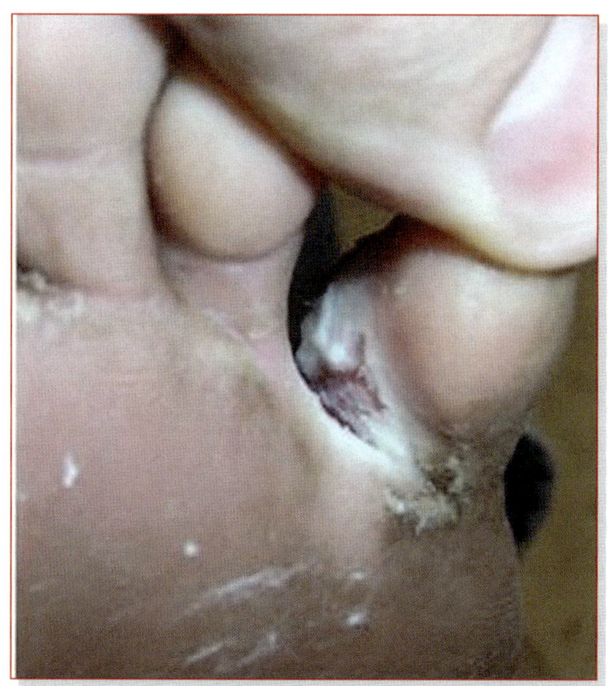

Athlete's foot

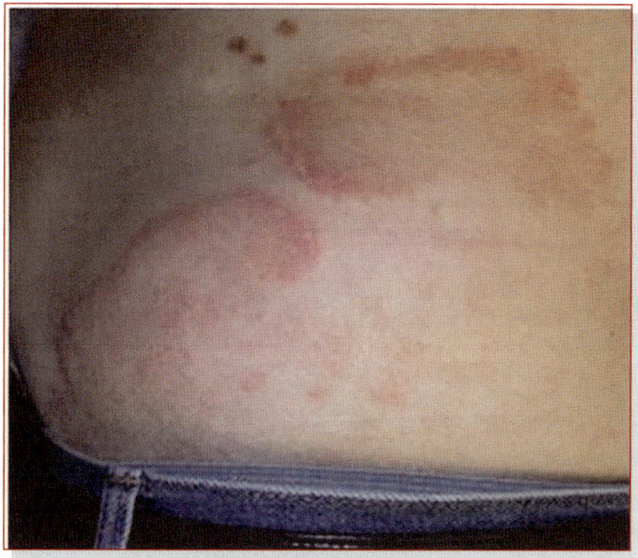

Ringworm on the back

Part I Medical Skin Conditions

Dry Skin

Dry skin may appear flaky and can be very itchy. Three factors that make dry skin worse include soap and water, cold air, and aging. For some patients it resolves naturally in the summer when skin retains its moisture better. Minimizing the amount of water and soap exposure may also help prevent the condition or keep it from getting worse. If soap is truly needed, Cetaphil and CeraVe liquid cleansers are recommended.

Moisturizers are the treatment of choice, and a variety are suitable, including Vaseline, Cetaphil, CeraVe, Lac-Hydrin, AmLactin, and urea creams. These products are available without a prescription. There is no best moisturizer; the one that feels best on your skin may be different than the one that feels best on another person's skin. Prescription-strength moisturizers, such as 40 percent urea cream, are also available, but these products may work no better than moisturizers available over the counter. Moisturizers work best when applied to damp skin immediately after bathing. Reapply them throughout the day as needed. If dry skin affects your hands,

Myths about Dry Skin

Patients routinely ask me what they can do about their dry skin. Often, however, when I examine them, I see that the problem is not dry skin—it's eczema or psoriasis. Eczema and psoriasis can look like dry skin, because affected skin flakes off. In fact, eczema and psoriasis are autoimmune conditions caused when the patient's immune cells mistakenly travel to the skin to fight an infection that doesn't exist. These immune cells cause skin flaking and sometimes an associated itch and rash. Treatment of eczema and psoriasis often requires topical corticosteroid creams, which remove immune cells from the patient's skin. Moisturizers help treat very mild eczema and psoriasis, but they are often inadequate by themselves.

Many patients also ask me what they can do for their dry scalp. Upon examination, I see flakes in the hair, but the problem is not dry scalp—it's seborrheic dermatitis. Seborrheic dermatitis can also appear as dry skin on the face and ears and is probably caused by the patient's immune response to a fungus living on the skin. The immune cells in the skin cause flaking and sometimes an associated itch and rash. Treatment of seborrheic dermatitis often requires an antifungal shampoo or cream that kills the fungus. Other treatments include shampoos that dissolve flakes or clear immune cells from the scalp. For more information, see the essays on "Seborrheic Dermatitis, Eczema, and Psoriasis" in Part I of this book.

apply a moisturizer after every hand wash. Finally, a humidifier in the home or workplace may alleviate the condition.

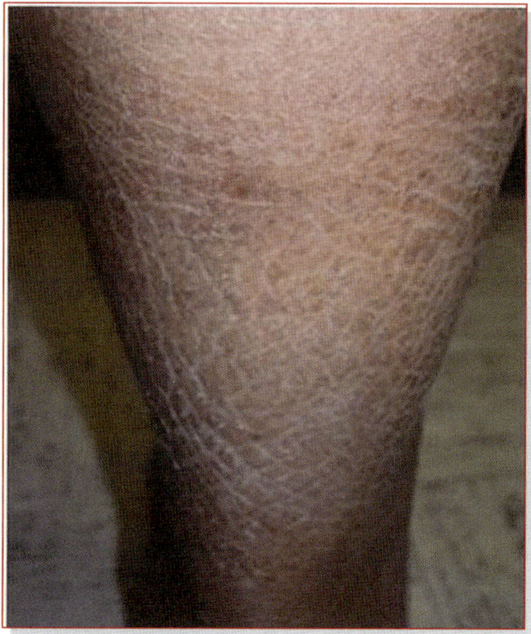

Dry skin

Dysplastic Mole (Dysplastic Nevus)

The subject of dysplastic (dis-plas´tik) moles is controversial. Dermatologists sometimes use the term *dysplastic mole* when they are referring to a mole that looks irregular to the eye. It may have several different colors, an irregular shape, or a large size. Your dermatologist may even remove a dysplastic mole to rule out the possibility of a melanoma, but interestingly, when a dysplastic mole is biopsied, the pattern of cells under the microscope may look completely benign. In this case, nothing else may need to be done. At other times, when a dysplastic mole is biopsied, the pattern of cells under the microscope may look abnormal. Pathologists often grade this abnormality on a spectrum from mild to moderate to severe. If the pattern of cells is moderately or severely abnormal under the microscope, the pathologist or dermatologist may recommend excising additional skin around the growth to make sure it is gone for good. If the pattern of cells is only mildly abnormal under the microscope, it is often acceptable to simply observe the area over time without removing additional skin.

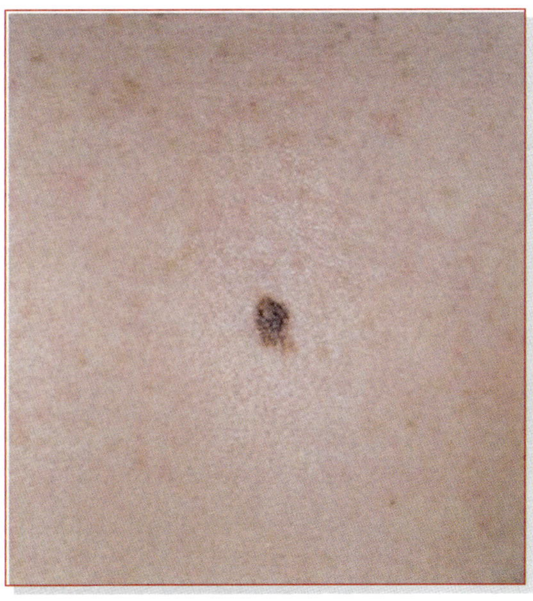

Dysplastic mole on the back

Highlights of a Dysplastic Mole Excisional Biopsy

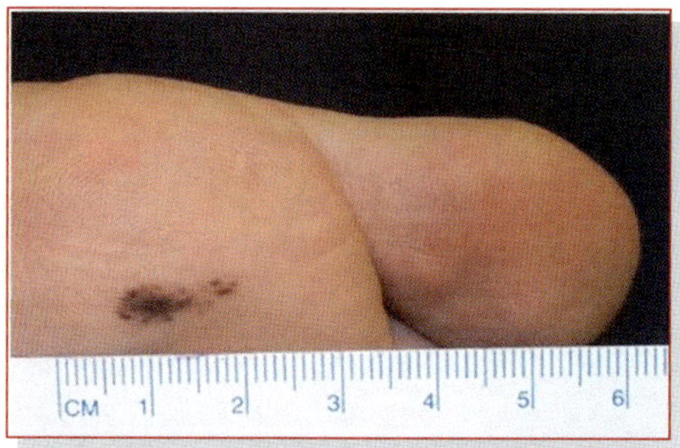

Dysplastic mole requiring an excisional biopsy to rule out melanoma.

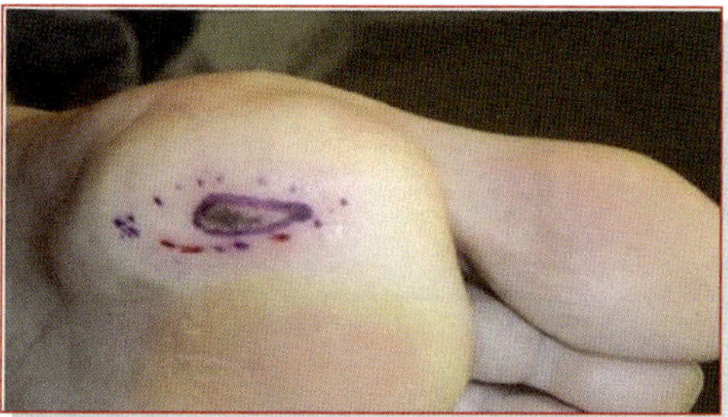

The perimeter of the dysplastic mole is outlined with a marking pen, and a small moat surrounding the mole is demarcated with a series of dots. The moat is shaped this way to permit an optimal closure. The dermatologist then injects lidocaine into the growth to numb the area. Finally, he excises the entire moat of skin demarcated by the dots.

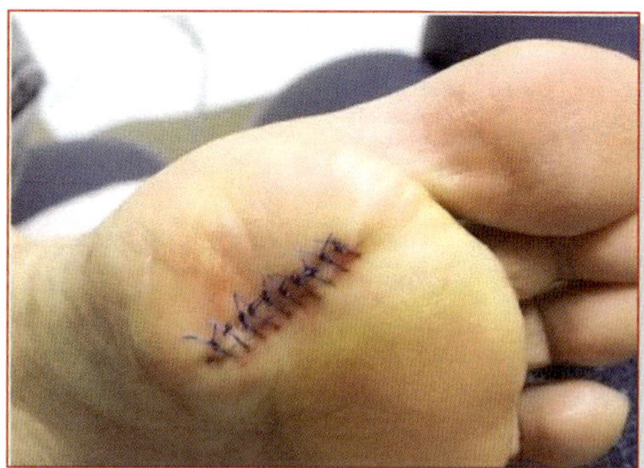

The dermatologist closes the site with sutures and removes them two weeks later.

Part I Medical Skin Conditions

Eczema

Eczema (ek´zĕ-mă) presents with itchy, pink, scaly patches of skin. It is an autoimmune condition caused when the immune system mistakenly sends T cells to the surface of the skin to fight an infection that does not exist. These T cells release chemicals that cause the redness and itching. The condition probably results from the combination of genes inherited from one's parents, since the genes are what largely program the immune system how to respond to different stimuli.

Eczema is also called atopic dermatitis when it presents in childhood in a characteristic skin distribution on the arms in front of the elbows and on the legs behind the knees. Atopic dermatitis typically resolves by adulthood. Eczema is treatable but not curable; therapies help suppress the condition but, if treatment is stopped, the condition may recur.

Washing over eczema with soap and water makes it worse, so minimize washing affected skin unless obviously dirty. When needed, use a gentle soap such as Cetaphil liquid cleanser, and avoid scrubbing affected skin with a cloth, brush, or sponge. Finally, avoid hot or very warm water when washing; try using cool water instead.

Cold, dry air in the winter makes eczema worse. Heaters that blow hot air into your room can also exacerbate the condition. For these reasons, a humidifier in the home or office, especially in the winter, may alleviate eczema.

Moisturizers are the treatment of choice for very mild eczema, and a variety are suitable, including Vaseline, Cetaphil, CeraVe, Aquaphor, Lac-Hydrin, AmLactin, urea creams, and others. These products are available without a prescription. There is no best moisturizer for everyone; the one that feels best on your skin may be different than the one that feels best on another person's skin. Moisturizers work best when applied to damp skin immediately after bathing. Reapply them throughout the day as needed.

The condition may not substantially improve with moisturizers. In this case, topical corticosteroid creams, including triamcinalone or clobetasol, are needed. These creams work by removing T cells from the skin and function best if applied immediately after bathing, when the skin is still damp. Apply them later in the day if needed—particularly before bedtime to avoid nighttime itching. Typically, eczema will resolve after several days at which point the T cells are out of the skin. Then, apply a bland moisturizer, such as Vaseline or Cetaphil, to help prevent the rash from coming back. The eczema could recur because corticosteroid creams don't cure the problem at the genetic level. If this happens, reapply the corticosteroid cream daily until you see improvement.

Corticosteroid creams applied daily for months with no breaks can slowly start to thin out the skin, resulting in a shiny and wrinkled look, and tiny blood vessels could appear in the skin. This side effect often resolves on its own after stopping the cream. Nevertheless, if you have used the cream daily for two weeks in a row, take a two-week break off the cream, or switch to weekend use only for a while before restarting it. Moisturize your skin during the break in therapy.

Other creams that work like corticosteroid creams but will not thin out the skin include Elidel (pimecrolimus cream) and Protopic (tacrolimus ointment). Elidel and Protopic are typically far more expensive to buy than clobetasol and triamcinalone creams, which are available in generic formulations.

Part I Medical Skin Conditions

More severe eczema not responding to corticosteroid creams may resolve with narrowband ultraviolet light type B phototherapy or oral medications, such as prednisone, CellCept (mycophenolate mofetil), Imuran (azathioprine), methotrexate, and cyclosporine. All of these treatments are discussed in Part II of this book.

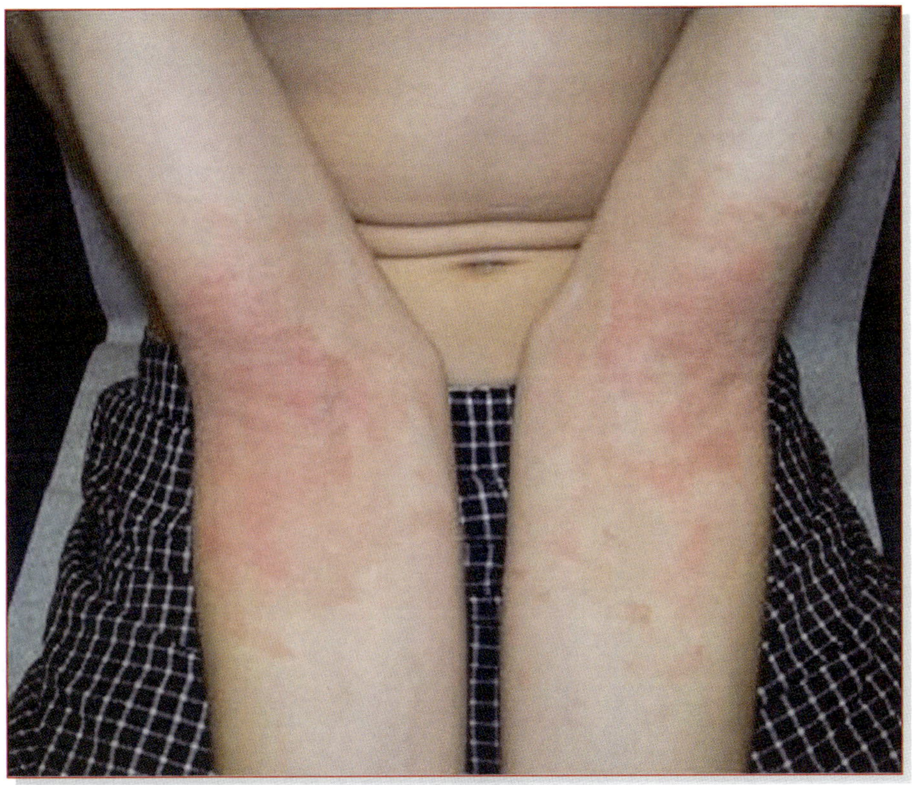

Classic eczema or atopic dermatitis

Erythema Nodosum

Erythema nodosum (er-i-thē′mă nodo′sum) presents as painful red lumps on the legs. It is an autoimmune condition caused when the immune system mistakenly sends immune cells to the skin of the legs to fight an infection that does not exist. The immune cells cause the pain and redness.

There are several reasons erythema nodosum may arise. In some cases, it results from a reaction to a new medicine, such as birth control pills or antibiotics. Discontinuing the medicine, in these instances, leads to resolution of the disorder. In other cases, infections such as *Streptococcal* infections, upper respiratory tract viral infections, *Mycoplasma* infections, or tuberculosis cause erythema nodosum. Treatment of the infection may resolve the skin condition in these instances.

Other autoimmune diseases, including inflammatory bowel disease and sarcoidosis, can cause erythema nodosum. In these cases, treatment of the underlying autoimmune disease helps alleviate the skin condition.

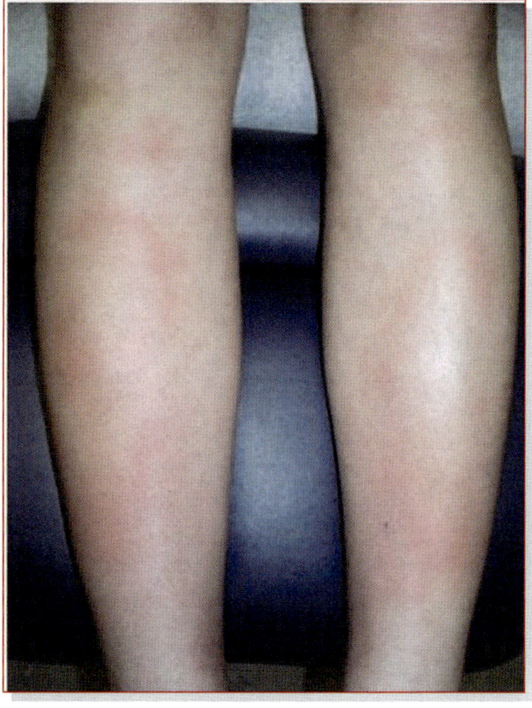

Erythema nodosum on the legs

In many circumstances, the cause of erythema nodosum is not found. Regardless of the cause, though, nonsteroidal anti-inflammatory medicines such as aspirin, ibuprofen, or naproxen help relieve pain, redness, and swelling. Potassium iodide is another medicine available for resistant cases.

Erythrasma

Erythrasma (er-i-thraz´mă) presents with reddish patches on the armpits and groin area that may or may not itch. Erythrasma is caused by bacteria called *Corynebacterium minutissimum*, which thrive on warm and moist skin. A chemical produced by the bac-teria reflects a fluorescent, coral color when exposed to a special lantern called a Woods lamp. Dermatologists frequently use a Woods lamp in the office to detect this color and confirm the diagnosis. Erythrasma is treated with prescription strength erythromycin gel twice a day for a few weeks. Once the condition clears, dry the affected skin after bathing. Then apply powder, such as Desenex or Zeasorb, to the same areas to help prevent recurrences. Desenex and Zeasorb powders are available without a prescription.

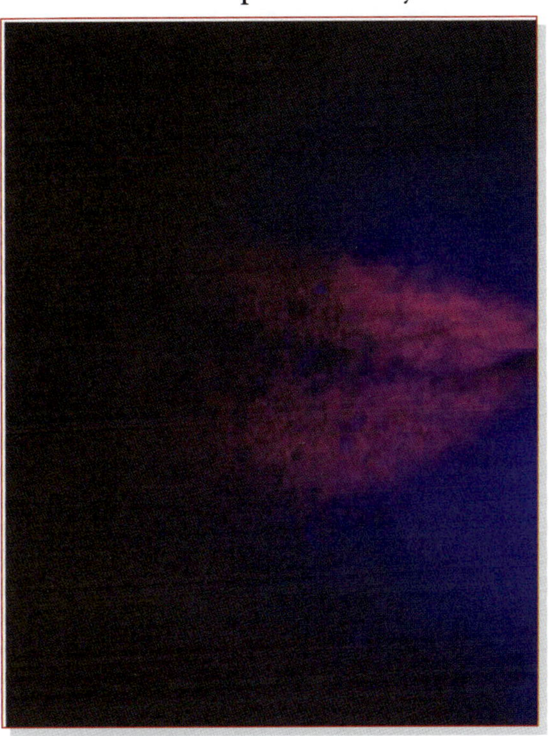

Coral fluorescence of erythrasma
of the armpit under a Woods lamp

Folliculitis and Abscess

Folliculitis (fŏ-lik-yū-lī´tis) means inflammation of the hair follicles. The condition usually presents as scattered pink bumps or pus-filled bumps on the skin. They can be itchy or painful. If the condition is left untreated, a very painful bump may arise on the skin, called an abscess (ab´ses) or boil. Folliculitis can be caused by bacteria, fungi, and viruses, but is probably most commonly caused by bacteria called *Staphylococcus*. This type of bacteria likes to live on warm, moist surfaces, such as in the nostrils, on the groin area, the buttock fold, the armpits, and under the breasts. Most of the time, *Staphylococcus* doesn't cause any problems and just sits there quietly. However, when it grows too much, or when it plants itself into a shaving nick, an infection may develop. For this reason, folliculitis most commonly arises on the buttocks, groin area, legs of women, beard area of men, armpits, and scalp.

Treatment of bacterial folliculitis may require oral antibiotics for approximately ten days. For folliculitis presenting on the legs or beard area, shaving habits may need to be changed. Generally, hair should be shaved in the direction the hair grows, down, with one stroke. Shaving against the grain or shaving with multiple strokes increases the likelihood of nicking the skin and should be avoided if possible. Finally,

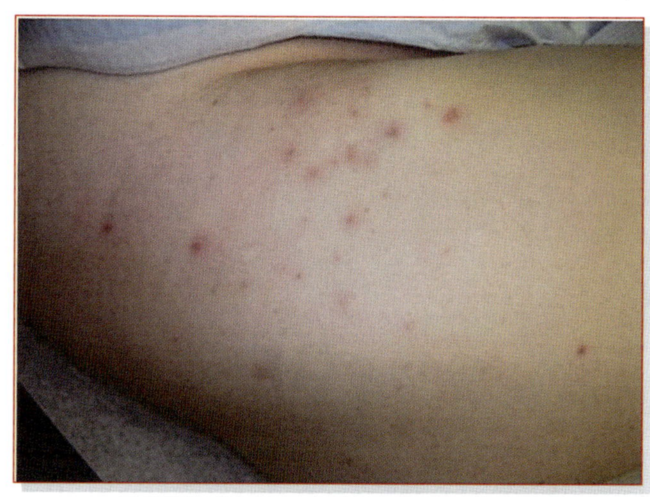

Folliculitis on the right thigh

Part I Medical Skin Conditions

treatment of an abscess requires draining the pus out, and antibiotics may be needed.

A bacterial culture can determine if you are colonized by *Staphylococcus*. If your nose is found to carry the bacteria, you should apply 2 percent mupirocin ointment with a Q-tip inside the nostrils twice a day for five days, and repeat this monthly. Doing so eliminates the bacteria from the nose and keeps it away. *Staphylococcus* carriers should also apply an antibacterial cleanser called Hibiclens to the groin area, buttock fold, armpits, and under the breasts in the shower, a few times a week. Using Hibiclens will help eliminate bacteria from these surfaces and keep it away. This cleanser can be purchased without a prescription from pharmacies and should not be applied around the eyes or ears. Together, mupirocin and Hibiclens may reduce the risk of developing folliculitis and other infections from *Staphylococcus* in the future.

Finally, *Staphylococcus* is contagious and easily spreads among members of the same household. *Staphylococcus* carriers should avoid sharing towels, washcloths, and sponges with other household members. In addition, they should consider having household members examined or questioned about their skin history. Household members should also consider using mupirocin and Hibiclens to prevent *Staphylococcus* from spreading again.

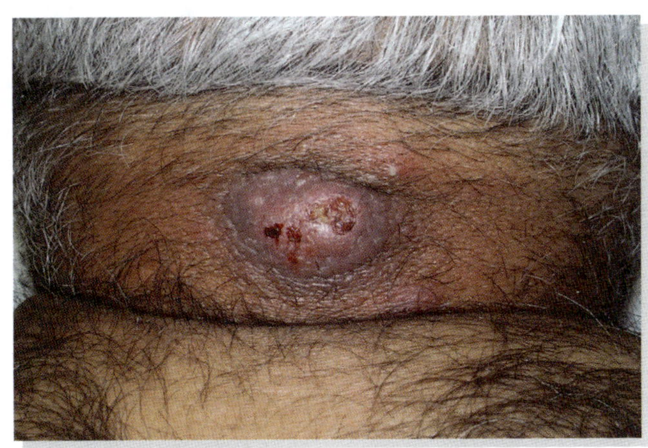

Abscess with surrounding folliculitis on the neck. *Staphylococcus aureus* caused this infection.

Granuloma Annulare

Granuloma annulare (gran-yū-lō´mă annula´re) presents as smooth-surfaced, raised rings on the skin. It is an autoimmune condition caused when the immune system mistakenly sends immune cells to the skin to fight an infection that does not exist. The immune reaction causes the circular bumps to form. It is not contagious or dangerous on its own. However, patients may develop diabetes with a higher than average incidence, so those displaying signs of diabetes, such as increased frequency of urination, may need a fasting glucose test.

In about half of observed cases, skin lesions can disappear within two years even without treatment. The spots may recur, however, sometimes in the exact same location

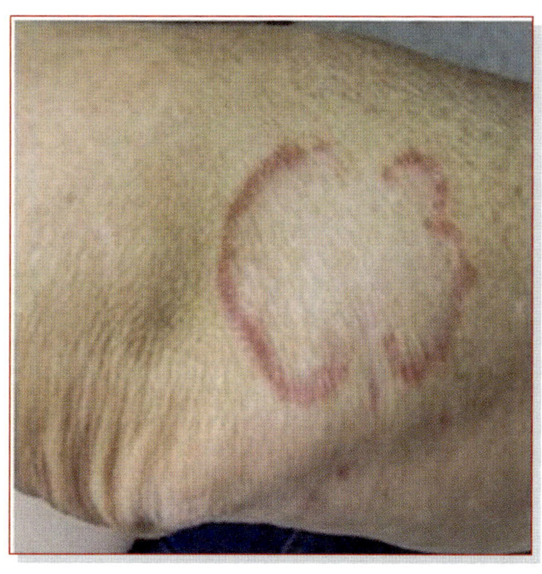

Granuloma annulare of the right arm

where they originated. If you desire treatment, the dermatologist can inject corticosteroids into skin lesions on a monthly basis until they fully resolve.

Granuloma Fissuratum

Granuloma fissuratum (gran-yū-lō´mă fish´ŭr-ătum) is a harmless condition that appears as a red bump or flat patch on the upper sides of the nose or on the crease between the ear and scalp. It results from eyeglass frames rubbing the nose or ears. Granuloma fissuratum resolves within a few months of replacing, adjusting, or discontinuing eyewear. Occasionally, a biopsy may be required to confirm the diagnosis and rule out the possibility of a skin cancer.

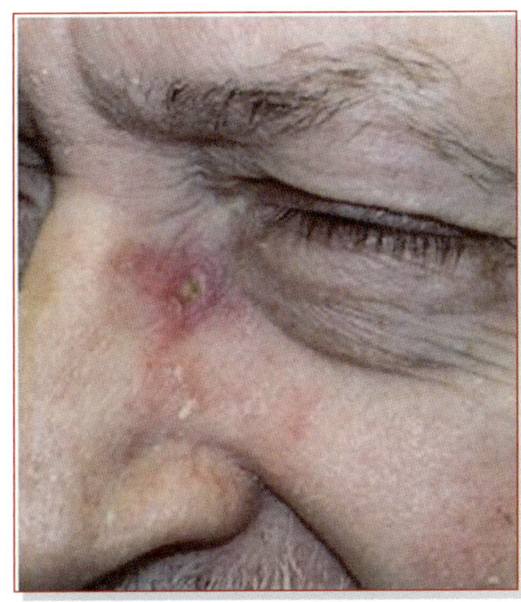

Granuloma fissuratum on the upper
nasal sidewall from tight-fitting glasses

Grover's Disease

Grover's disease is named for the physician Ralph Grover. It typically presents in adulthood as very itchy bumps on the chest, abdomen, and back. Bumps are often pink with a tiny, crusted surface. Doctors have not determined what causes Grover's disease. It is neither infectious nor contagious. Sometimes a biopsy is required to confirm the diagnosis and rule out other conditions, such as folliculitis. Grover's disease tends to persist, often for several months.

Heat and sweating may make Grover's disease worse. Therefore, try to wear loose-fitting clothing and stay cool. Topical corticosteroid creams such as triamcinalone or clobetasol help control the itch, but they are not considered a cure because if application is stopped, the spots may come back. These creams work best if applied to damp skin after showering. After your skin improves significantly, stop the corticosteroid cream and try to maintain your improvement with either Cetaphil moisturizer or Sarna lotion, which are available without a prescription. If the bumps come back, simply reapply the corticosteroid cream daily until they disappear again.

Applying corticosteroid creams daily for multiple weeks with no break can start to thin out the skin, resulting in a shiny and wrinkled look, and tiny blood vessels could appear in the skin. For this reason, if you have used the cream daily for two weeks in a row, take a two-week break or switch to weekend use only for a while before restarting it. Moisturize your skin or apply Sarna lotion during this break in therapy. Sarna lotion treats itch and is available from pharmacies without a prescription.

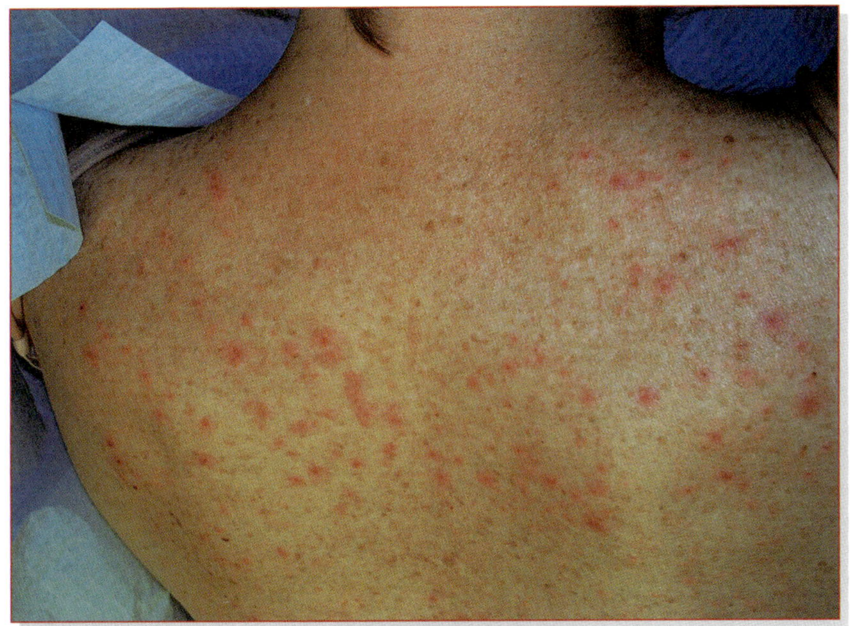

Grover's disease on the back

Herpes

Herpes presents as itchy or painful fluid-filled bumps on an inflamed, pink base of skin. Breakouts last about a week and typically resolve even with no treatment. Herpes is common and may arise anywhere on the body. It is caused by a virus that is transmitted by physical contact. Sometimes the virus infects skin without any visible signs. During this dormant phase, the virus is still contagious and can infect others unknowingly. Stress and other illnesses can cause herpes in the dormant phase to erupt into visible bumps. Sometimes it erupts for no reason at all. After a week or so, the bumps dry up and fall off. Unfortunately, herpes never really goes

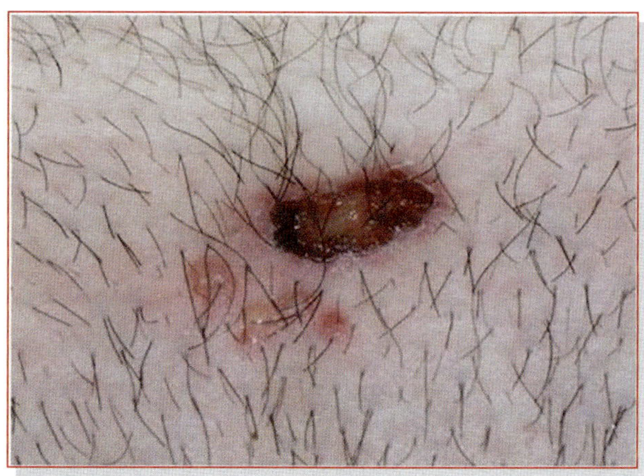

Fluid-filled and crusted bumps from herpes

away after this but returns to the dormant phase.

Treatments should be initiated immediately after you notice herpes arising on your skin, because if you wait more than a few days, the medicines will probably fail. The goal of therapy is to reduce the duration of breakout. Herpes outbreaks around the mouth can be treated with Abreva, which is available without a prescription. Apply it immediately upon recognizing the breakout, five times a day, until lesions resolve. Zovirax (acyclovir), Valtrex (valacyclovir), and Famvir (famciclovir) are other prescription-strength medicines for herpes.

Patients suffering from multiple breakouts every year may elect to take Valtrex on a daily basis throughout the year to reduce the frequency and severity of breakouts. The daily use of Valtrex may also reduce the risk of transmitting herpes in its dormant phase to one's partner. Condoms help prevent the transmission of herpes too.

Hidradenitis Suppurativa

Hidradenitis suppurativa (hi´drad-ĕ-nī´tis sŭp´yŭr-ă-tiv´ă) usually presents in adolescence as painful draining boils in the armpits and groin. Doctors are not certain what causes hidradenitis, but the condition may result from a problem with the apocrine glands, which are concentrated under the skin of the armpits and groin area. Many patients are concerned that hidradenitis is an infection and contagious, but it actually is not. In many people, hidradenitis persists for years.

Since many patients with this condition also suffer from obesity, treatment may begin with weight loss. Cleansing the affected areas with Hibiclens in the shower may also help by removing bacteria that accumulate in the area. Antifungal powders, such as Desenex or Zeasorb powder, applied after showering, will also help keep the affected areas dry and fungus-free. Hibiclens, Desenex, and Zeasorb can all be purchased without a prescription.

Painful areas are often drained and cultured to rule out an infection. Early lesions are injected with a corticosteroid called triamcinalone to reduce redness, swelling, and pain, and to decrease the likelihood that they will drain out. Other medicines available for hidradenitis include oral antibiotics, Soriatane (acitretin), Remicade (infliximab), and monthly treatments with an ND-YAG laser. Finally, excising the affected skin can afford long-lasting relief in some patients.

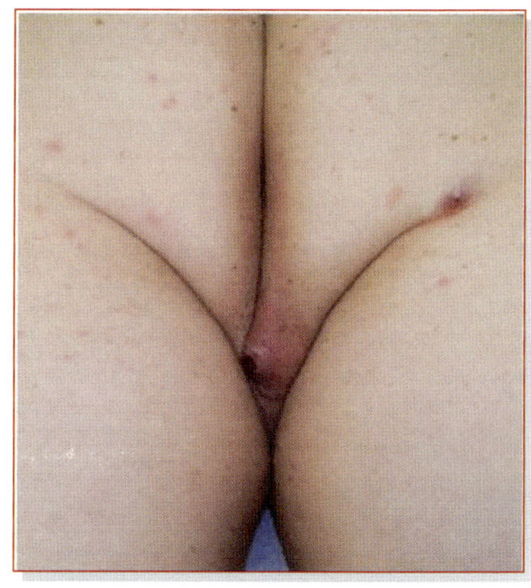

Hidradenitis suppurativa on the buttocks

Hives

Hives are pink, smooth, itchy bumps that disappear in less than twenty-four hours and then reappear in other places. In some patients, swelling in or around the mouth and eyes may also develop—a condition called angioedema. Hives is an autoimmune condition caused when the immune system mistakenly sends immune cells and immunoglobulins to the skin to fight an infection that does not exist. These immune cells and immunoglobulins are what cause the rash. Patients with hives may develop other genetically related autoimmune conditions such as thyroid disease, diabetes, rheumatoid arthritis, and pernicious anemia.

Some patients develop hives due to skin exposure to something in the environment, such as water, sun, cold, or even a specific clothing fabric. Hives can also result as a reaction to medicines, such as angiotensin-converting enzyme inhibitors for hypertension (enalapril), nonsteroidal anti-inflammatory medicines (aspirin, ibuprofen, or naprosyn), and opioids (morphine and oxycodone). Interestingly, infections in the body can also cause hives. Finally, hives may result from foods. If you think this is the case, keep a diary of what you eat and when hives arise to see if a food could be causing them. Unfortunately, despite everything that will be done to find and eliminate the cause of hives, in some people the cause is never found.

The course of hives is different in everybody. Sometimes hives resolve within a few weeks

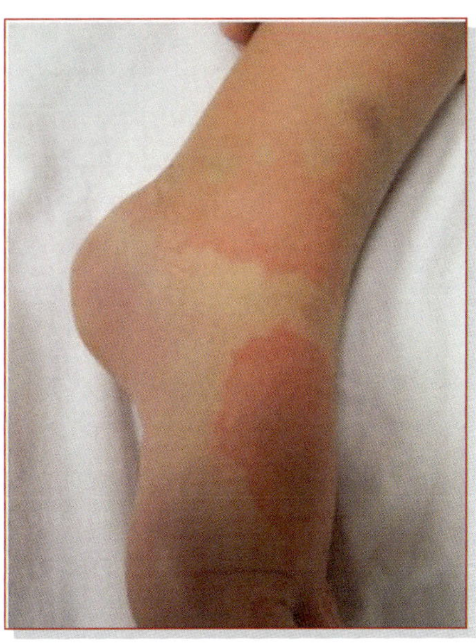

Hives

and never recur. Other patients suffer recurrences whenever exposed to a trigger. A few people live with hives continuously. Unless the cause of your hives is found and eliminated, the duration of your condition may be unpredictable.

Treatments for hives are designed to decrease the frequency and severity of breakouts. Unfortunately, they are not cures because, if treatment is stopped, the hives could come back. Even when the treatments are working, breakthrough hives may arise.

Calamine lotion, Sarna lotion, and Aveeno oatmeal creams and baths are soothing anti-itch treatments available without a prescription. Reducing your exposure to stress, preventing yourself from overheating, and drinking less alcohol may also help. If the cause of your hives is uncertain, consider trying a low pseudoallergen diet for three weeks by avoiding artificial colorings, preservatives, and natural salicylates. Document your response in a food diary.

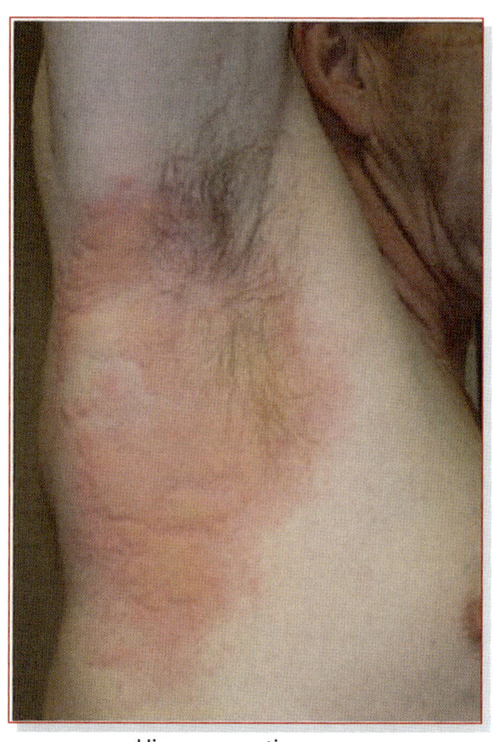

Hives presenting as a
reaction to an Under Armour outfit

Antihistamine drugs are the treatment of choice for hives. A nonsedating antihistamine, such as 180 mg Allegra (fexofenadine), 10 mg Claritin (loratadine), or 10 mg Zyrtec (cetirizine) is often prescribed for the morning. If your hives do not respond, you may require a higher dose. A sedating antihistamine is also often prescribed at bedtime to help you sleep. Benadryl (diphenhydramine), Atarax (hydroxyzine), and doxepin are examples of sedating antihistamines. Start by taking a small dose of sedating antihistamine to make sure you don't sleep through the alarm clock the next morning. If the initial dose doesn't help, you may require a higher dose. Taking too high of a dose, however, could cause side effects such as constipation, urine retention, dry mucous membranes, and dizziness. Patients failing to respond to antihistamines may require narrowband ultraviolet light type B phototherapy or cyclosporine. See Part II of this book for more information about these treatments.

Hyperhidrosis

Hyperhidrosis (hī′per-hī-drō′sis) presents with excessive sweating of the hands, feet, armpits, or other surfaces. Patients often report they can only wear clothes of a certain color or fabric in order to conceal their sweating. Other patients feel awkward shaking hands with others due to sweaty palms. It is unclear exactly what causes hyperhidrosis, but many treatments are available.

Antiperspirants containing aluminum chloride represent the first-line treatment of hyperhidrosis of the armpits. Certain Dri is one such product available without a prescription. Dry-Sol is an alternative that requires a prescription. Apply these products at bedtime. Dry off sweaty areas first, and then apply the antiperspirant. In the morning, wash off the product. Repeat this process for a few days until you see results. Once results are seen, continue to apply the product every few days, just frequently enough to maintain your improvement. You may find that you only need to apply it every other day, every third day, or every fourth day to maintain results—everybody is different.

Iontophoresis is another treatment for hyperhidrosis of the hands and feet, but not the armpits. With iontophoresis, the hands or feet are placed in pans filled with water for about twenty minutes, while a very mild electric current effectively shuts down the sweat glands. This is repeated every other day for five to ten days or until sweating improves. Once it works, you still need maintenance sessions, but treatments once a week to once every four weeks may suffice to maintain your improvement. Iontophoresis units are available with a doctor's prescription from R.A. Fischer Company.

Iontophoresis is not appropriate for hyperhidrosis of the armpits, and it sometimes fails to work for the hands and feet. In these cases, Botox (botulinum toxin) may be an appropriate treatment. Botox is injected into the skin and works by shutting down the sweat glands. Results are seen within a few days and can last six months or more. Usually, twenty injections are required per armpit. Surprisingly, it is not very painful, but applying a lidocaine cream thirty minutes before treatment reduces any discomfort you might experience. LMX 4 and LMX 5 are lidocaine creams available without a prescription.

When hyperhidrosis fails to respond to conventional treatments, is widespread, or affects the face and scalp, pills may be needed. For example, glycopyrrolate is a pill that reduces sweating from the entire skin. Possible side effects include dry mouth, dry eyes, difficulty with urination, constipation, palpitations, and blurry vision. Patients are started on a low dose, such as 1 mg daily, and the dose is slowly escalated until results are seen. Once side effects are encountered, the dose is lowered until they resolve.

Intertrigo

Intertrigo (in-ter-trī´gō)presents as inflamed patches of skin under the chest, in the groin, in the buttock crease, in the armpits, or between the fingers. These skin folds are warm and moist and therefore attract a variety of infectious agents. Bacteria such as *Streptococcus, Corynebacterium,* and *Pseudomonas,* and fungi such as *Candida,* dermatophytes, and *Malassezia* are common causes of intertrigo. Sometimes intertrigo is not due to an infection; for example, psoriasis can cause intertrigo.

Typically, a combination of creams, including triamcinalone cream, ketoconazole cream, and erythromycin gel, is used to treat intertrigo. Weight loss may also help clear up intertrigo. If psoriasis is causing the condition, however, a single corticosteroid cream such as triamcinalone or a nonsteroidal anti-inflammatory ointment such as Protopic (tacrolimus) is the recommended treatment.

Once the rash clears up, try an antifungal powder such as Desenex or Zeasorb to prevent recurrence. These powders are available without a prescription. Finally, restart your prescription cream or creams if the condition recurs.

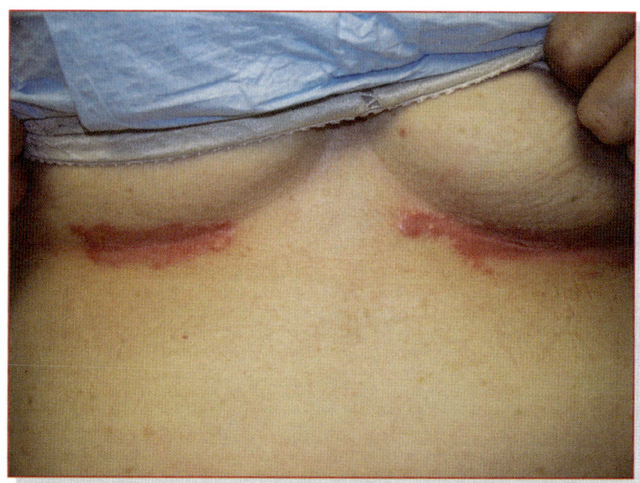

Intertrigo under the chest due to psoriasis. This is not an infection.

Keratosis Pilaris

Keratosis pilaris (ker-ă-tō´sis pila´ris) is a harmless skin condition usually arising on the arms and sometimes the thighs and cheeks. It presents as tiny bumps, often on the skin of eczema patients. Sometimes the skin can appear red around the bumps. Technically, the condition results from plugged hair follicles—but doctors don't know exactly why this happens.

Keratosis pilaris is treatable but not curable; therapies help suppress the condition, but if treatment is stopped, the condition may recur. Applying 12 percent Lac-Hydrin or AmLactin cream twice daily helps smoothen and flatten out the bumps. Redness around the bumps sometimes responds to hydrocortisone cream. AmLactin cream and hydrocortisone cream are available without a prescription.

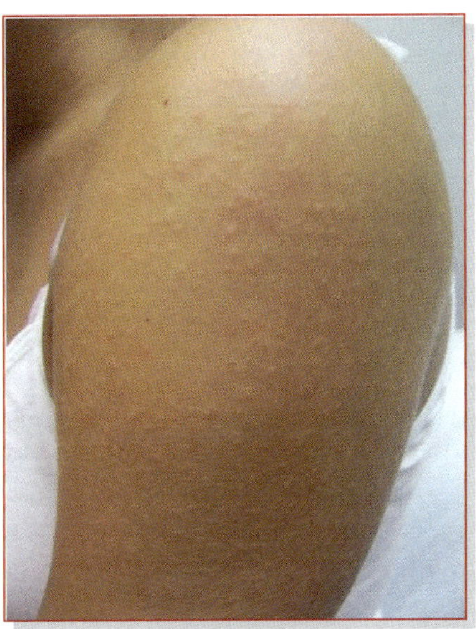

Keratosis pilaris.
It looks like acne, but it isn't.

Lentigo

A lentigo (len-tī´gō) is a brown, flat spot that sometimes arises from sun exposure. It can also be called an age spot, liver spot, freckle, or a sun spot. Lentigines are harmless and do not need to be removed. However, if you dislike their appearance, they may be treated. Once you commit to a treatment, avoid excessive sun exposure to help the treatment work and to prevent the development of new spots. For advice on sun protection, see the beginning of the essay "Skin Aging: Prevention and Treatment" in Part I of this book.

If you have only one lentigo, spraying the spot with liquid nitrogen may be the simplest treatment option. Liquid nitrogen is extremely cold and works by causing a small, localized frostbite over the lentigo. You will feel some stinging and burning when the dermatologist freezes the lesion, but the discomfort is tolerable and temporary. No special skin care is required after treatment. The lentigo forms a little scab over the next two weeks and falls off. Healthy skin will replace the lentigo.

The freezing effect of liquid nitrogen could cause a fluid-filled blister, which resolves in a few days without treatment. There is also a small chance you may need a second freeze to remove the lentigo. Therefore, if a spot has not fallen off by one month after treatment, return for a touch-up session. Finally, treated skin could look somewhat darker or lighter than surrounding skin for months after treatment.

Hydroquinone cream can also lighten lentigines when applied twice daily. This cream takes approximately two months to fully kick in, so if results are not seen by this time point, return to the dermatologist for reexamination.

Retinoid creams, such as tretinoin cream, are also useful for the treatment of lentigines. These creams also take approximately two months to reach their maximum potency, so if results are not seen by

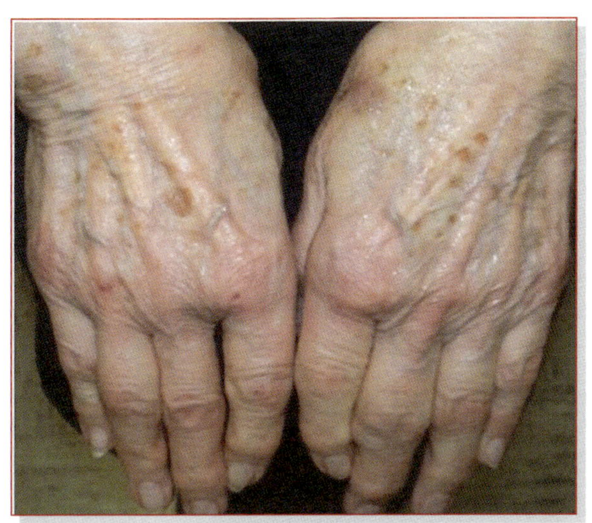

Lentigines of the hands

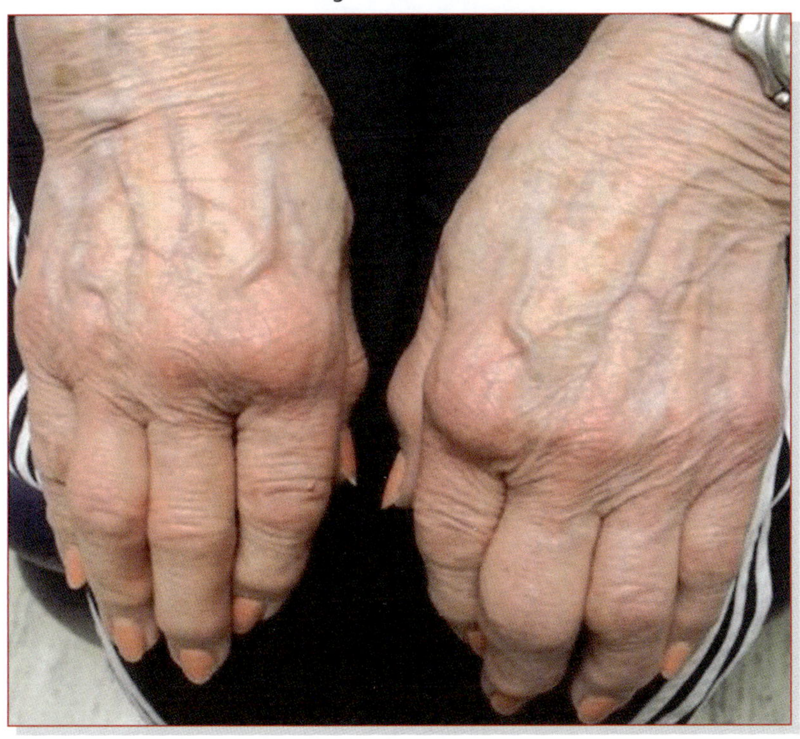

Clearance of lentigines after one session of intense
pulsed light, the routine use of hydroquinone cream, and sunscreen

this time point, return to the dermatologist. Place a small, pea-sized amount of cream on your index fingertip, then rub the cream into your fingers, and finally apply a thin layer over the spots, but avoid the eyelids. Use tretinoin cream at nighttime because sunlight deactivates it.

If it causes dryness and peeling, try applying a smaller amount. Placing a moisturizer like Cetaphil facial moisturizer right over the tretinoin cream at night and throughout the day will also reduce dryness and peeling. Finally, cutting back the frequency of application will reduce irritation. Tretinoin cream may still work if used every third or fourth night. Other retinoid creams are also available without a prescription, but they may not work as well.

Multiple lentigines are also treatable with glycolic acid or trichloroacetic acid chemical peels. Finally, a field of lentigines may respond to intense pulsed light treatments. With this technique, a beam of light is shined on the skin and targets pigment within the lentigines. One to three treatments may be required for clearance. See Part III of this book for more information about chemical peels and intense pulsed light.

Leukocytoclastic Vasculitis

Leukocytoclastic vasculitis (lū′kō-sī-tō-klas-tik vas-kyū-lī′tis) presents as reddish or purplish patches, most commonly on the lower legs. Vasculitis is an autoimmune condition caused when the immune system mistakenly sends neutrophils to the skin to fight an infection that does not exist. The resulting inflammation makes blood vessels in the skin burst, which creates the purple colored rash. In many cases, only the skin is involved, but in other instances the neutrophils travel to and affect the joints, kidneys, intestines, heart, lungs, or even brain.

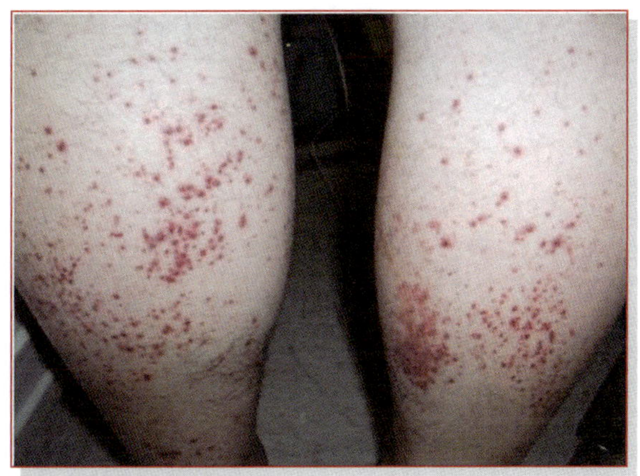

Leukocytoclastic vasculitis on the legs

There are several reasons vasculitis may arise. In some cases, it results from a reaction to a new medicine. The most common medications causing vasculitis include allopurinol, antibiotics, nonsteroidal anti-inflammatory medications (aspirin, ibuprofen, and naprosyn), and sulfonamides (Bactrim, furosemide, glyburide, and hydrochlorothiazide). Vasculitis arising as a drug reaction typically starts one to three weeks after a person starts taking a drug and stops soon after he or she discontinues the medication. In other instances, infections may cause vasculitis. Typical infections include urinary tract infections, pneumonia, and hepatitis. Treatment of the infection may resolve the vasculitis in this case.

Connective tissue diseases, such as rheumatoid arthritis and lupus, and other types of diseases, such as Wegener's granulomatosis, Churg-Strauss disease, microscopic polyarteritis, cryoglobulinemia, and inflammatory bowel disease can also cause vasculitis. In these circumstances, treatment of the underlying disease helps eliminate the rash.

Finally, cancer can cause vasculitis. For this reason, make sure you are up to date with your age-associated recommended cancer screenings, including a colonoscopy, Pap smear, mammogram, or prostate examination. A workup for patients with blood cell count abnormalities may also be warranted to rule out blood cell cancers.

Treatments for vasculitis work by removing neutrophils from the skin. Prednisone is commonly prescribed for vasculitis and works rapidly. Other medications such as dapsone, colchicine, pentoxifylline, Imuran (azathioprine), or methotrexate may also resolve the condition. See Part II of this book for more information about some of these treatments.

Lichen Planus

Lichen planus (lī´ken pla´nus) may present on the skin, in the mouth, on the head, or on the nails. On the skin, lichen planus is characterized by tiny purple bumps that often itch. It can also appear in the mouth as white, wispy, colored patches on the inside of the cheeks. On the scalp, lichen planus causes inflamed patches of skin and hair loss. Finally, it can present with degeneration of the nails.

Lichen planus is an autoimmune condition caused when the immune system mistakenly sends T cells to the skin, mouth, scalp, or nails to fight an infection that does not exist. These T cells release chemicals that cause the redness and itching. Doctors are not certain exactly what causes lichen planus, but in some patients, an underlying infection with hepatitis C may be responsible. In other patients, lichen planus arises due to a reaction to a new medicine. Some medicines that more commonly cause it include angiotensin-converting enzyme inhibitors (captopril), beta blockers (metoprolol), gold, nonsteroidal anti-inflammatory medicines (aspirin, ibuprofen, and naprosyn), and penicillamine.

The course of lichen planus is unpredictable. A majority of patients with lichen planus on the skin only will have their condition spontaneously resolve within a year. Oral lichen planus can be more persistent. In any case, you may desire treatment to make you more comfortable.

Topical corticosteroid creams such as clobetasol and triamcinalone can be applied daily on the rash. These creams work by removing T cells from the skin, and they function best if applied to damp skin immediately after bathing. Apply the cream daily until the purplish rash resolves at which point the T cells are out of the skin. You may now be left with a brown stain in the skin that will resolve on its own over a period of months. Corticosteroid creams do not remove this brown stain.

Applying corticosteroid creams daily for weeks with no breaks can start to thin out the skin, resulting in a shiny and wrinkled look, and tiny blood vessels could appear in the skin. Therefore, if you require the cream for fourteen consecutive days, take a two-week break or switch to weekend-only use for a while before restarting it.

If the condition is more widespread, you may benefit from narrowband ultraviolet light type B phototherapy. Treatments are administered two or three times a week for about two months. Sessions are then slowly tapered off. If light treatments are not appropriate or do not work, or if the condition affects your nails or hair, you may benefit from systemic treatment. Griseofulvin, Soriatane (acitretin), Plaquenil (hydroxychloroquine), cyclosporine, and methotrexate may successfully resolve lichen planus. See Part II of this book for more information about these treatments.

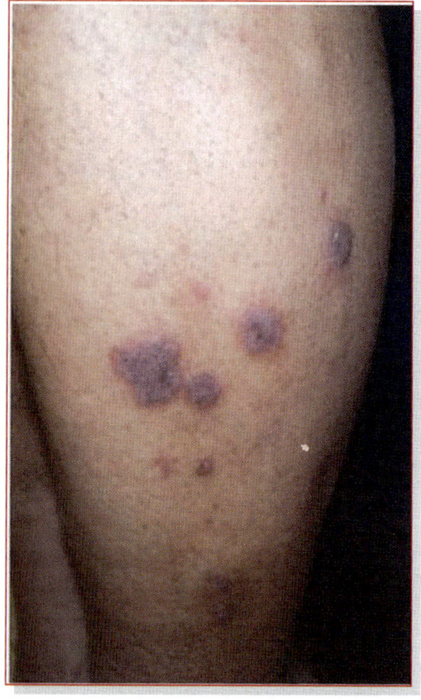

Lichen planus of the
skin in a patient with hepatitis C

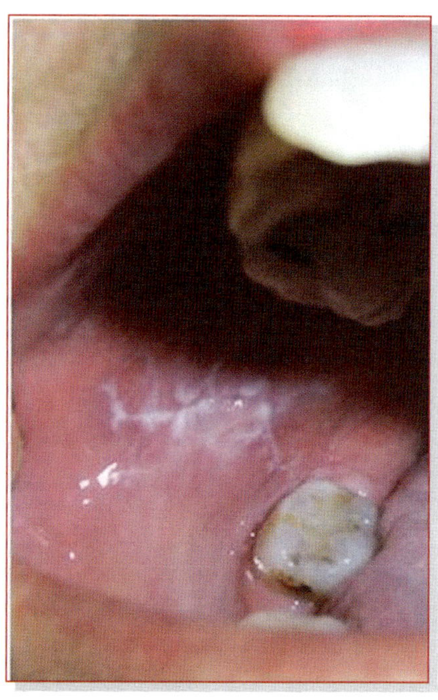

Lichen planus of the mouth

Lichen Simplex Chronicus

Lichen simplex chronicus (lī´ken sim´plex chronicus) is a fancy name for thickened, itchy skin. It most commonly arises on the back of the neck, legs, arms, and the genitals. The skin assumes a leathery appearance due to constant rubbing and scratching. Patients have developed a habit of scratching their skin, and they can't stop. Interestingly, the skin loses the leathery appearance when the rubbing stops. The treat-

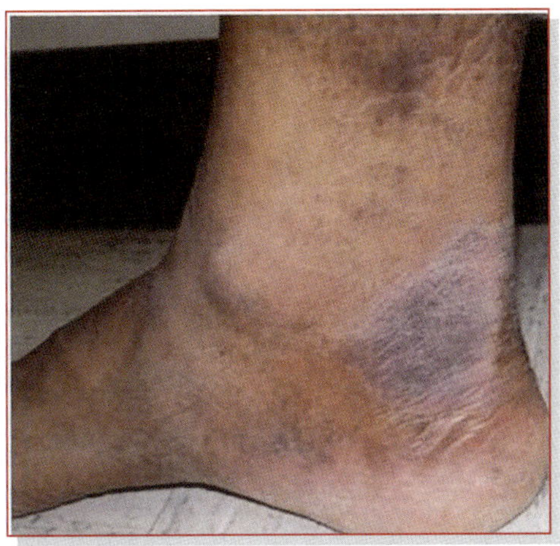

Lichen simplex chronicus

ment is, therefore, to do everything in your power to stop scratching. The dermatologist's job is to find any underlying skin disease that causes itch, such as eczema, and treat it effectively. Therapies include corticosteroid creams, such as triamcinalone or clobetasol, or a corticosteroid tape, such as Cordran tape, which is placed over the leathery skin and replaced when it falls off. Other patients may benefit from taking a low dose of a sedating antihistamine pill such as Benadryl (diphenhydramine), Atarax (hydroxyzine), or doxepin once or twice daily.

Lipodermatosclerosis

Lipodermatosclerosis (lip´ō-der´mă-tō-sklĕ-rō´sis) presents as painful, firm, reddish, warm areas on the lower legs. It is not an infection and does not respond to antibiotics. In many cases, patients with lipodermatosclerosis are mistakenly treated with antibiotics for an infection called cellulitis; some are even sent to the hospital for this purpose.

According to one hypothesis, lipodermatosclerosis may result from poorly functioning leg veins. Properly working leg veins return blood from the feet back to the heart. When these veins stop working well, blood pools in the legs, allowing irritating chemicals to leak into the surrounding skin. The immune system mounts a reaction to these irritating chemicals, leading to lipodermatosclerosis.

Lipodermatosclerosis is difficult to treat and requires patience. First, keep your legs elevated–preferably to the level of your heart–whenever you are sitting down. This makes it easier for poorly functioning veins to return blood to the heart. Second, consider wearing support hose or compression stockings during the day, which, again, help return pooling blood in the legs back to the heart.

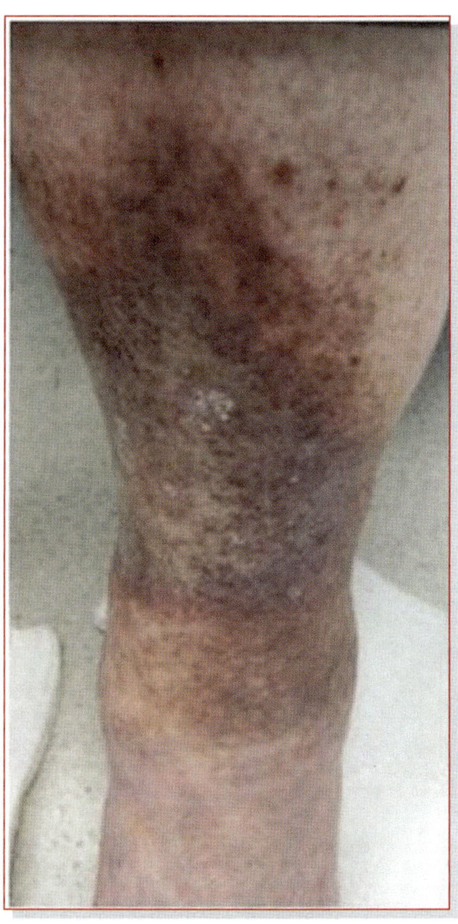

Lipodermatosclerosis

Part I Medical Skin Conditions

Jobst is a brand of support hose and compression stockings available without a prescription.

Other treatments include weeks of physical therapy using an ultrasound machine applied to the legs. A drug called Trental (pentoxifylline) and prescription anabolic steroids may also resolve lipodermatosclerosis. Finally, poorly functioning veins can be treated by a vein specialist.

Lipoma

Lipomas (li-pō´măs) present as soft lumps underneath the skin. When the tissue of a lipoma is examined under a microscope, normal fat cells are typically seen. Hence, lipomas can be thought of as overgrowth of fat in a local area. Dermatologists have not found the cause for this process. Once discovered, a lipoma could stay the same size, or it could grow larger—one cannot predict ahead of time.

If it does not bother you, a lipoma need not be removed. However, if it does bother you, the lipoma may be excised. The dermatologist first injects the lipoma with lidocaine to numb the area and then removes the tissue with a scalpel in a painless manner. He or she then closes the site with stitches, which need to be removed, typically in two weeks.

Part I Medical Skin Conditions

Highlights of a Lipoma Excision

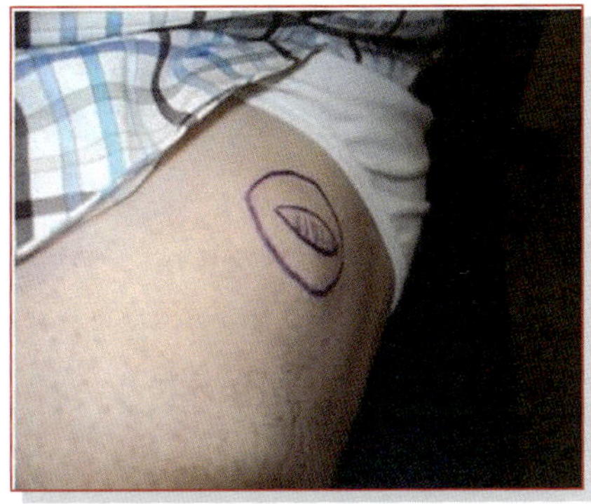

Lipoma marked out before surgery.

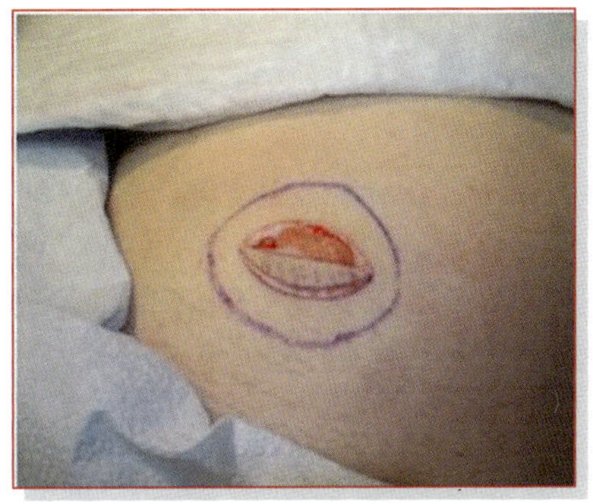

Lipoma fat bulges out
after the first incision is made.

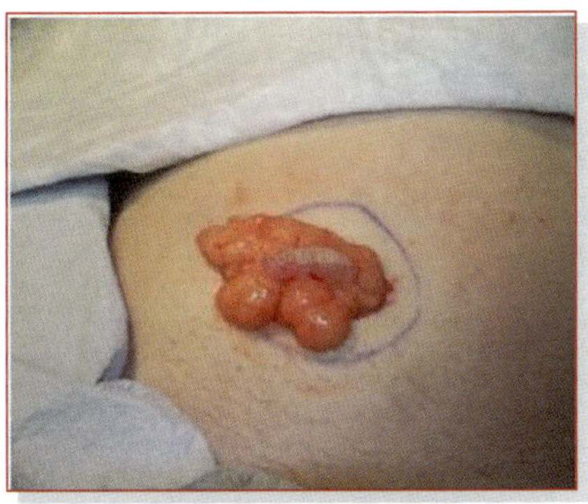

Lipoma fat completely
exposed by dissection.

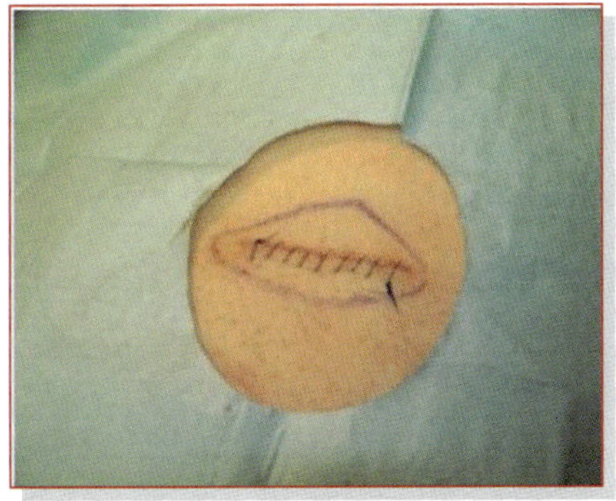

Closure with sutures after lipoma removal.

Lupus

Lupus (lū´pŭs) is an autoimmune condition caused when the immune system mistakenly sends T cells and immunoglobulins to the skin to fight an infection that does not exist. These T cells and immunoglobulins cause the lupus rash. For some patients, the cause of lupus remains unknown, but it can sometimes arise as an immune reaction to a newly started medicine. Lupus can potentially affect different parts of the body, but in some people it just affects the skin or scalp. For example, some lupus patients develop a rash and nothing else. Others develop joint pain, low blood cell counts, kidney disease, lung disease, and central nervous system conditions, such as seizures. Many treatments exist for lupus, but if they are stopped, the condition may recur.

Patients should avoid intense sun, because sunlight, even the amount that travels through windows, can make skin lupus worse. Sunlight could even trigger lupus to start affecting the internal organs. Patients with some hair loss should use a spray sunscreen to treat the scalp, because a lupus rash on the scalp can

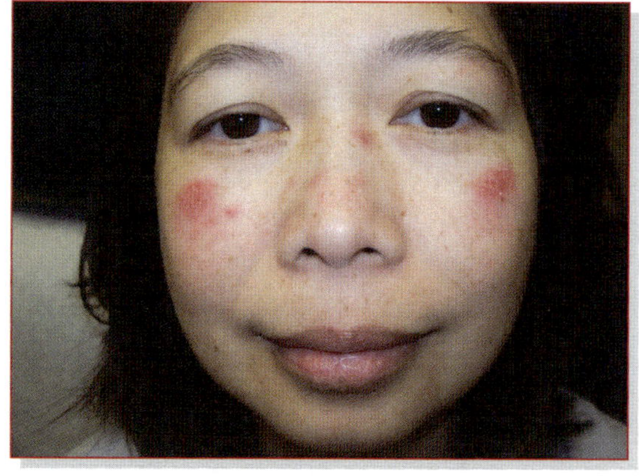

Lupus affecting facial skin

cause hair loss. For advice on sun protection, see the beginning of the essay "Skin Aging: Prevention and Treatment" in Part I of this book.

Treatment for skin lupus involves topical corticosteroid creams, such as triamcinalone or clobetasol, or nonsteroidal anti-inflammatory creams, such as Elidel (pimecrolimus cream) or Protopic

Part I Medical Skin Conditions

(tacrolimus ointment). Scalp lesions may require a corticosteroid foam, such as Luxiq (betamethasone valerate) or Olux (clobetasol), or corticosteroid injections into the scalp. Finally, resistant cases may respond to prednisone, Plaquenil (hydroxychloroquine), and steroid-sparing drugs, such as Imuran (azathioprine) and CellCept (mycophenolate mofetil). Steroid-sparing drugs are typically administered with prednisone to help lower the prednisone dose needed. See Part II of this book for more information about these treatments.

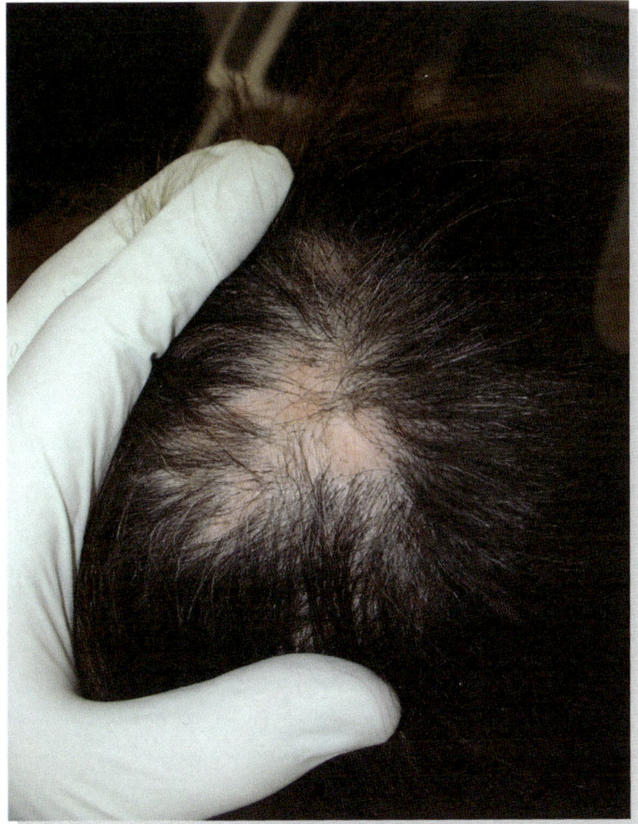

Lupus affecting the scalp

Melanoma

Melanoma (mel´ă-nō´mă) is a serious form of skin cancer that usually arises as a black patch or bump. It may arise from the damaging effects of sunlight over many years; however, a melanoma may arise anywhere on the body, not just on the face or other sun-exposed surfaces.

If melanoma is found early and has not spread roots into the dermis, it is called melanoma in situ and can often be removed without serious repercussions. However, if melanoma is allowed to grow deep roots before it is removed, it is more likely to spread around the body and be difficult to cure.

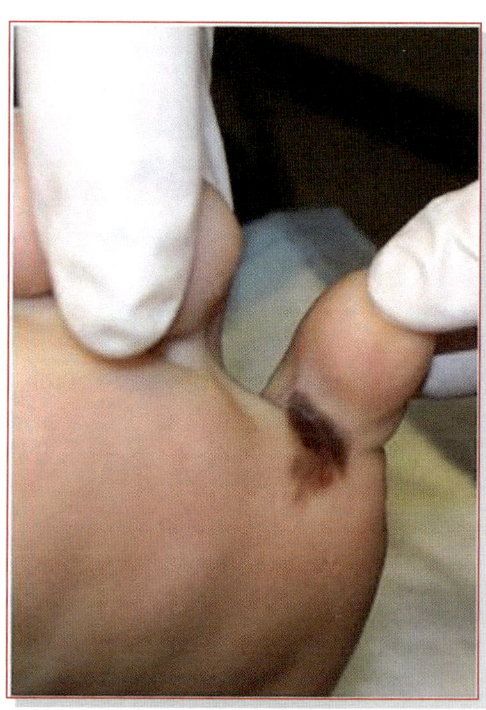

Melanoma in situ of
the left fifth toe web space

The standard treatment for melanoma is an excision. The dermatologist first injects lidocaine around the melanoma to numb the area. He or she then removes the melanoma and a moat of skin around it with a scalpel. The size of the moat removed depends on the size of the melanoma.

Melanoma patients need a full skin examination to make sure nothing is hiding anywhere else on the skin. The lymph nodes also need to be examined because advanced melanoma could spread there.

A procedure called a sentinel lymph node biopsy is available for patients with larger melanomas. With this test, the lymph nodes around the cancer are removed and examined microscopically to see if the melanoma is present within the nodes. The results of this test may give a sense of how serious the condition is. Blood work, X-rays, CT scans, and PET scans are usually reserved for cases in which there is evidence that the melanoma may have spread to other areas.

Melanoma patients could develop a recurrence, or second skin cancer, and therefore require a full skin examination on a regular basis far into the future. It is also important to limit sun exposure to help prevent the development of additional skin cancers. For advice on sun protection, see the beginning of the essay "Skin Aging: Prevention and Treatment" in Part I of this book.

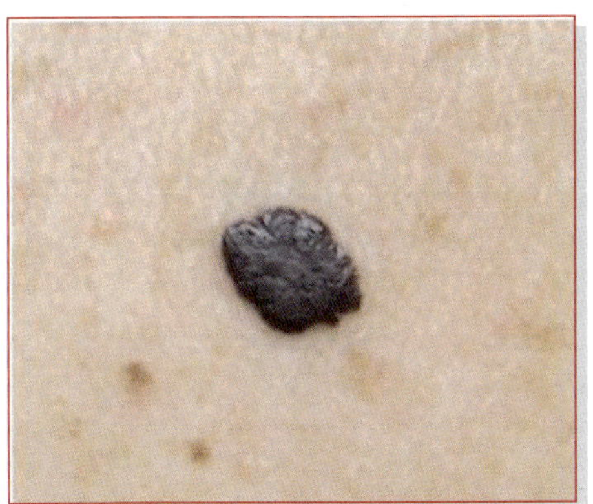

Melanoma that has grown roots down into the dermis. It measured one centimeter along its longest axis.

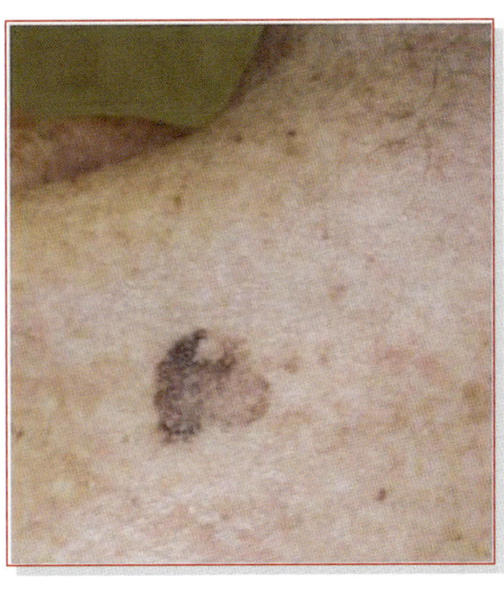

Melanoma in situ of the left upper back.

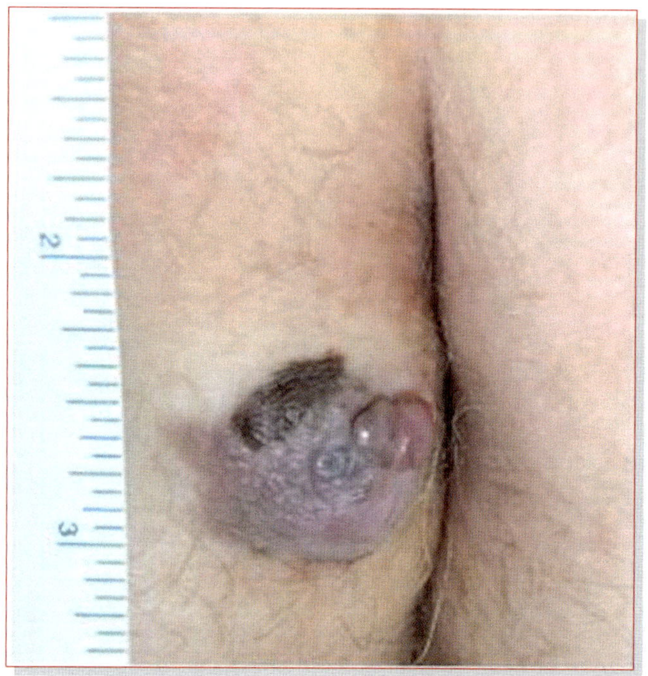

Melanoma presenting as a large, pink nodule on the left buttock. Not all melanomas are black. This photo also illustrates that a melanoma can arise anywhere on the body, even in places that receive minimal to no sun. Finally, the case demonstrates that melanomas can arise as collision lesions. What does that mean? When the patient shown above first presented, a shave biopsy was performed on a portion of the nodule, and the pathologist issued a report characterizing the lesion as a harmless mole. I asked the patient to return for another biopsy to confirm the diagnosis. This time the entire nodule was shaved off and sent to the pathologist, who issued a report describing the lesion as a very large melanoma. A melanoma and a mole can arise within the exact same area, by coincidence. When this happens, the hybrid growth is called a collision lesion. In this case, the first biopsy picked up only the mole portion, and the second biopsy was needed to confirm the diagnosis of real importance.

Highlights of a Melanoma Excision

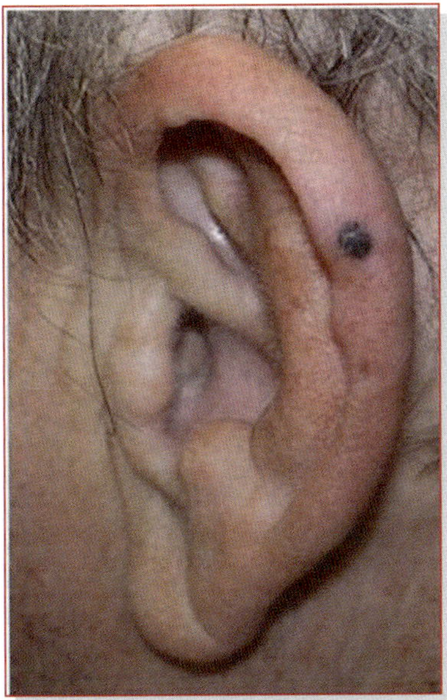

Melanoma.

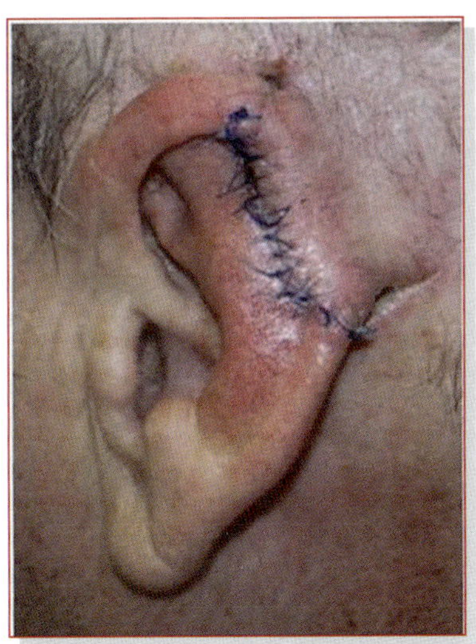

Once the melanoma was excised, a skin flap was placed over the surgery site to allow the area to heal.

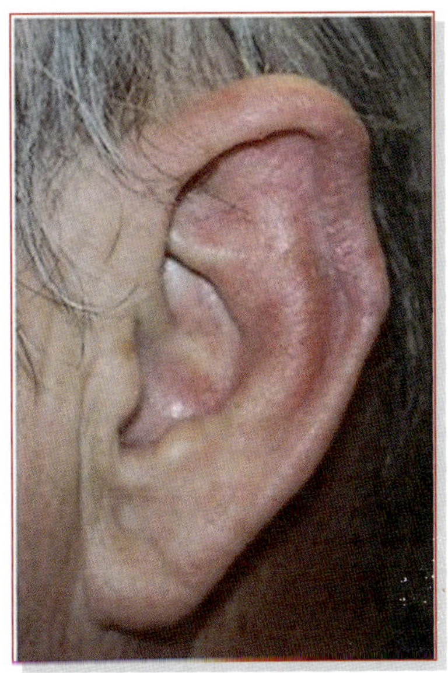

Final cosmetic result.

Melasma

Melasma (mĕ-laz´mă) presents as dark patches of skin, often on the forehead and cheeks. It may arise from hormone changes since it frequently presents around the time of pregnancy or during the use of oral contraceptives. Melasma comes in two varieties: superficial and deep. Some patients have both types of melasma at the same time. The deep type of melasma may not respond well to treatments. Examination of the skin with a special lantern called a Woods lamp can help determine which type of melasma is present.

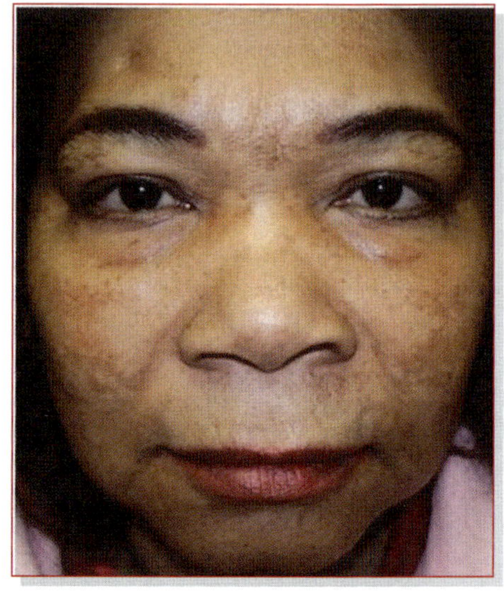

Melasma

Melasma can last for years, and treatment is often difficult, because sunlight makes it worse and reverses the benefits of treatment. For advice on sun protection, see the beginning of the essay "Skin Aging: Prevention and Treatment" in Part I of this book.

After committing to avoiding intense sun, melasma treatment may be initiated. Insurance may not cover the cost of therapy because it is considered cosmetic, not medical. Hydroquinone cream is a generic medicine helpful for melasma. Apply a small amount to the dark patches twice daily. If results are not seen after two months, a stronger hydroquinone cream or other treatment may be needed. Additional pharmaceuticals for melasma include tretinoin cream, which one should apply at night, Finacea (azaleic acid gel), which one should apply twice a day, Kojic acid, which can be mixed into hydroquinone cream by a compounding pharmacy, and glycolic acid peels, which may be repeated every few weeks. See Part III of this book for more information about chemical peels.

Part I Medical Skin Conditions

Mole (Nevus or Beauty Mark)

Moles (mōlz) are very common harmless growths that most often appear brown, but they may be tan, black, pink, or even reddish. They typically start out as flat, brown round spots. Later they can lose their color, become raised, and appear like soft, dome-shaped bumps. Although moles are by themselves harmless, patients with many moles—fifty or more—may be at risk for skin cancer later in life.

Moles begin developing in childhood, and the number of moles typically peaks around age thirty. Excessive sun exposure may cause moles to form, and applying sunscreen daily may reduce the number of moles arising in childhood. Staying out of intense sun and avoiding sunburns may also reduce the number of moles that develop.

Sometimes it is very difficult to tell the difference between a mole and skin cancer, particularly melanoma. In general, moles tend to have one uniform color and a symmetrical shape; you could draw a line down the middle of one and it would appear the same on both sides. On the other hand, skin cancers like melanoma may have more than one color, such as black and brown, and an asymmetrical shape. On average, skin cancers also tend to be larger than moles and grow faster.

Examine your moles on a monthly basis and stay alert for any change in size, shape, or color. See a dermatologist if any moles start changing size, shape, or color. Also consider seeking advice if a newly arising growth looks much different from your other spots. Your dermatologist may use a dermatoscope to look at moles with magnified, polarized light, which gives him, or her, an excellent view. He or she may also biopsy any questionable moles.

Moles can be removed for cosmetic purposes, but insurance may not cover the cost. Moles can either be shaved off or excised. If moles are shaved off, only the protruding surface is removed.

Many patients prefer this technique because it is quick, and they will no longer feel or see the dome-shaped bump. Shaving a mole will leave a small circular mark where the mole was, but in many cases the appearance of this mark fades with time, and many patients prefer the small mark to the appearance of the original mole. After shaving the lesion, however, some mole cells may be left under the skin, and the mole recurs in about 20 percent of cases.

Excising the mole will remove it permanently. Excising the mole involves removing skin all the way down to fat, all around the mole. Typically, the surgical site must be closed with stitches, and a small linear scar remains. The scar often looks increasingly better with time.

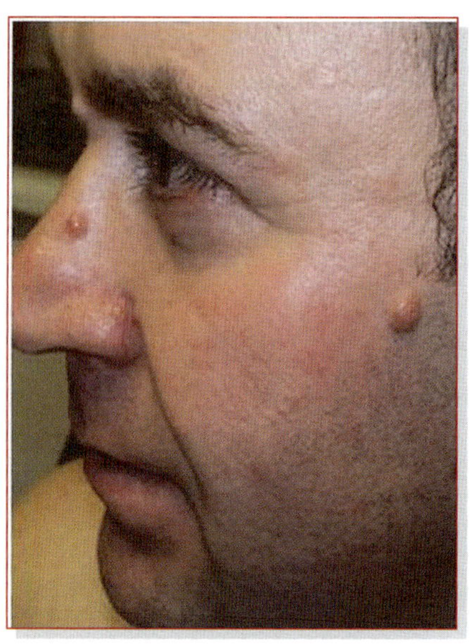

Multiple moles on the face. Each lesion is symmetrical and of one color, assuring the dermatologist that they are harmless growths.

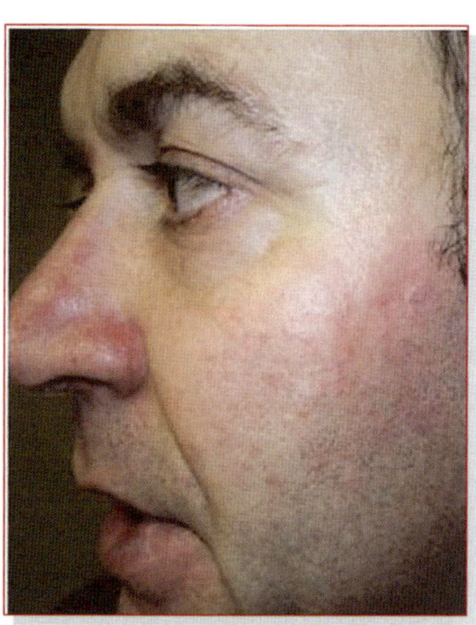

Cosmetic result after mole removal with the shave technique.

Molluscum Contagiosum

Molluscum contagiosum (mo-lŭs´kŭm contagio´sum) is a common skin disorder seen primarily in children, characterized by small pink bumps, some of which have a central dimple. They are caused by a virus that finds its way into the skin and makes the infected cells keep dividing until a visible bump arises. Patients may inadvertently acquire the virus by contact with someone else who has it. Molluscum can also be transmitted by scratching one location, which picks up the virus under the fingernails, and then scratching somewhere else, which deposits the virus elsewhere. If left alone, the lesions may resolve on their own. However, they may persist for years and spread if not treated.

Dermatologists treat lesions by spraying them with ice-cold liquid nitrogen, which causes a temporary, localized frostbite over the molluscum. Patients will feel some stinging and burning when the lesions freeze, and sensitive children especially may benefit from the liberal application of numbing cream to the area 30 minutes prior to treatments to reduce discomfort. LMX5 is a brand of lidocaine numbing cream available without a prescription. No special skin care is required after treatments. The molluscum form little crusts over the next two weeks and fall off. Healthy skin will replace the bumps.

The freezing effect of liquid nitrogen could cause a fluid-filled blister, which resolves without treatment in a few days. There is also a small chance you may need

> ### Myths about Molluscum Contagiosum
>
> **"Molluscum contagiosum does not need to be treated because it will go away on its own."**
>
> While this may be true for some patients, especially if they wait long enough, untreated molluscum multiplies on the skin of other patients. Moreover, it spreads to other people in the meanwhile. It is impossible to identify which course the molluscum will take for any given patient. In addition, the condition is easy to treat when only a few skin lesions are present, but cases are much more difficult to handle when dozens and dozens of molluscum arise. Why not nip the problem in the bud when it first arises?

a second freeze to remove the molluscum. Therefore, if a spot has not fallen off by one month after treatment, return for a touch-up session. Finally, treated skin could look somewhat darker or lighter than surrounding skin for months after treatment.

Aldara (imiquimod cream) is also used to treat molluscum. This cream stimulates your immune system to attack skin cells infected with the molluscum virus. Apply a small amount of cream to each spot at bedtime, and cover them with a small adhesive bandage. Then fold up the medicine packet and save any unused cream in the refrigerator for later use. Wash off the cream in the morning. Repeat this process three to five nights per week for a few months or until the skin clears. Treated bumps may look red and inflamed. That is expected and may signify that the treatment is working. If the treated spots become painful, stop the cream for a while and consider restarting it with less frequent applications when feeling better.

Dermatologists may also prescribe Condylox gel for molluscum contagiosum. It works by inhibiting rapidly dividing cells. Apply a small amount to the bumps twice daily for three consecutive days—for example, Monday, Tuesday, and Wednesday. If lesions have not resolved by Sunday, apply the gel twice daily for three consecutive days again. Three-day application sessions can be repeated two more times if needed. If no improvement is seen at that point, return to the dermatologist for reevaluation.

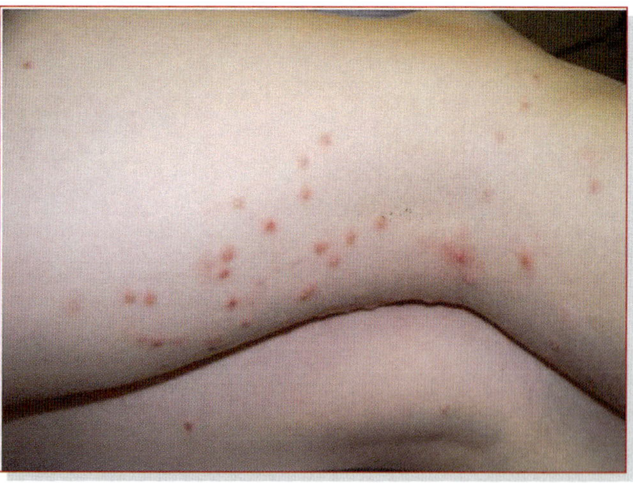

Molluscum contagiosum

Mycosis Fungoides

Mycosis fungoides (mī-kō′sis fungoi′des) is a type of skin cancer that usually presents as pink patches on Caucasian patients and tan patches on African American patients. Mycosis fungoides can look exactly like eczema and is occasionally mistaken for it. However, eczema is commonly reported as itchy, and mycosis fungoides often does not itch. Eczema and mycosis fungoides can even look similar under the microscope, and multiple skin biopsies are sometimes needed to differentiate between the two conditions.

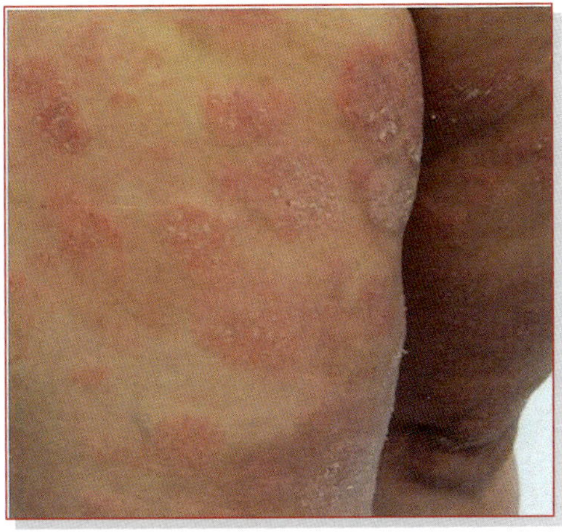

Mycosis fungoides on the thighs

When mycosis fungoides presents as flat patches on just a limited area of skin, it is typically not life-threatening and responds well to treatment. In very advanced cases, however, mycosis fungoides presents as firm, painful, skin lumps that may or may not bleed. This is called the tumor stage of mycosis fungoides and is serious.

The early, patch stage of mycosis fungoides may be treated with corticosteroid creams, such as clobetasol. Other topical therapies for the patch stage include mechlorethamine and carmustine. These topical remedies are applied consistently until the skin clears and then are used less frequently to maintain clearance. Mycosis fungoides may come back if treatments are stopped for too long. In this case, patients may need to restart therapy.

Topical remedies are generally safe, but patients on mechlorethamine may have an increased risk of developing skin cancer after long-term use. In addition, patients on carmustine must have periodic blood tests to monitor their blood cell counts, which can sometimes drop during treatment.

Narrowband ultraviolet light type B phototherapy and another type of light treatment called PUVA are available for patch stage mycosis fungoides that is very widespread or fails to respond to topical treatments. See Part II of this book for more information about phototherapy. Finally, patients with the tumor stage of mycosis fungoides may need to see an oncologist for consideration of chemotherapy.

Notalgia Paresthetica and Macular Amyloidosis

Notalgia paresthetica (nō-tal´jē-ă paresthet´ica) presents with severe itching of the upper midback. Sometimes a brown patch appears in the area, but at other times the skin looks completely normal. Doctors are not certain exactly why this condition arises, but some believe that patients may have an increased number of nerves in the area. There is no known cure for notalgia paresthetica, but treatments are

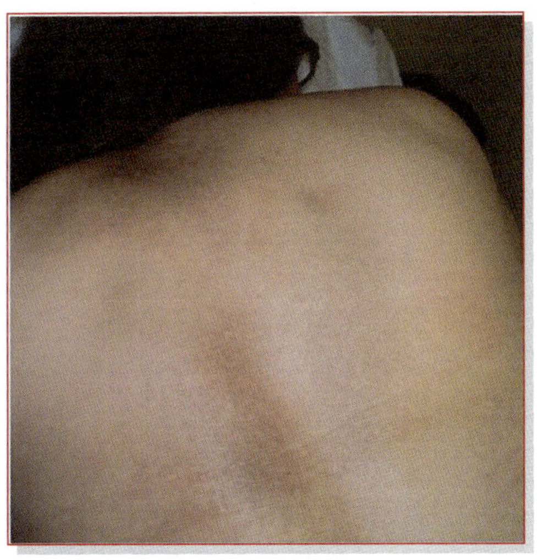

Notalgia paresthetica

available. For example, topical capsaicin cream applied five times daily for one week, followed by three times daily for three to six weeks, may help. Capzasin is a brand of capsaicin cream available without a prescription. Lidocaine cream applied several times a day may also reduce itch. LMX 4 and LMX 5 are brands of lidocaine cream available without a prescription. Finally, prescription-strength corticosteroid creams, such as clobetasol and triamcinalone, applied once or twice daily may alleviate itch.

Macular amyloidosis (mak´yū-lăr am'i-loy-dō´sis) is similar to notalgia paresthetica. Both conditions present with extreme itchiness in the upper midback. Sometimes a patch of brown skin appears in the area. A skin biopsy may confirm the diagnosis by demonstrating increased amyloid protein in the skin. No one knows what causes macular amyloidosis, but constant rubbing may aggravate or even cause the condition. Therefore, patients should avoid rubbing the area. Corticosteroid creams, such as clobetasol or triamcinalone, may also relieve the itch.

Onycholysis

Onycholysis (on-i-kol´i-sis) arises when a fingernail or toenail dislodges from the nail bed underneath. In some cases, it may be difficult to identify the cause, but a variety of processes can disrupt the bond between the nail plate and nail bed.

For example, chemicals that irritate the skin of the nail bed or that cause an allergy of the nail bed may cause onycholysis on the fingernails. Once chemicals break the bond between the nail bed and nail plate, future exposure to the same chemicals or even to water should be avoided by wearing gloves or finger cots. Finger cots are little rubber sleeves that cover the fingertips, and they can be purchased from local and online pharmacies.

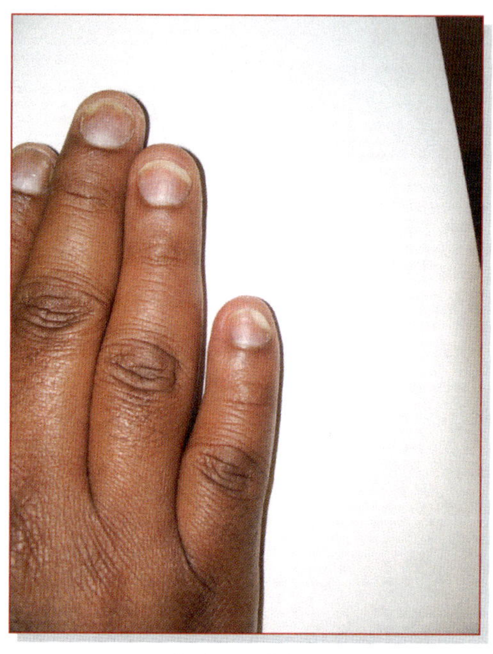

Onycholysis of the right pinky fingernail due to psoriasis

Physical trauma to the nails while performing one's occupation or engaging in hobbies may also cause onycholysis. For example, dishwashers and gardeners are at risk for onycholysis of the fingernails, and athletes and dancers are at risk for onycholysis of the toenails.

Certain drugs are known to cause onycholysis by making the nail bed sensitive to sunlight. Sunlight, in turn, damages the bond between the nail plate and nail bed. Medicines implicated in onycholysis include angiotensin converting enzyme inhibitors

Part I Medical Skin Conditions

(captopril), beta blockers (propranolol), hydrochlorothiazide, nonsteroidal anti-inflammatory medicines (aspirin, ibuprofen, indomethacin, and naprosyn), oral contraceptives, and quinolone antibiotics.

Onycholysis has also been associated with systemic diseases, including anemia, thyroid disease, lupus, and scleroderma. Skin diseases such as lichen planus and psoriasis may also cause onycholysis. Finally, pregnancy may lead to onycholysis for unknown reasons.

Treatment of onycholysis takes a long time and is difficult. First, clip your nails back as far as possible to prevent any overhanging nail plate from catching on objects and further pulling the nail plate off. Also, limit chemical and water exposure to the nails by wearing light cotton gloves under heavy-duty vinyl gloves when performing wet work or handling chemicals. Heavy-duty vinyl gloves are available at paint stores and pharmacies. Nails can also be kept dry with finger cots. In addition, protect your nails from cold weather by wearing lined leather gloves. Finally, avoid wearing high heels and narrow-tipped shoes that could worsen onycholysis of the toenails.

Fungal colonization under the nail plate may aggravate onycholysis or delay healing of the nails, so consider applying the antifungal cream Loprox (ciclopirox olamine) twice a day for at least twelve weeks to the affected nails. Antifungal pills such as fluconazole (150 mg, taken weekly) can also be considered. Finally, patients taking a drug that could cause onycholysis should consider finding a substitute medicine or should wear opaque nail polish and apply sunscreen directly to nails.

Paronychia

THE CHRONIC FORM

Paronychia (par-ō-nik´ē-ă) means "inflammation around the nail." Aggressive manicures, biting nails, and picking at cuticles may all cause paronychia. These activities separate the nail plate from the surrounding nail folds, forming a pocket in which water can get trapped. Subsequently, organisms such as *Candida* (a type of fungus) and bacteria proliferate in the moist pocket. An immune response to these organisms leads to redness and swelling, and if the condition lasts for more than six weeks, the condition is called chronic paronychia.

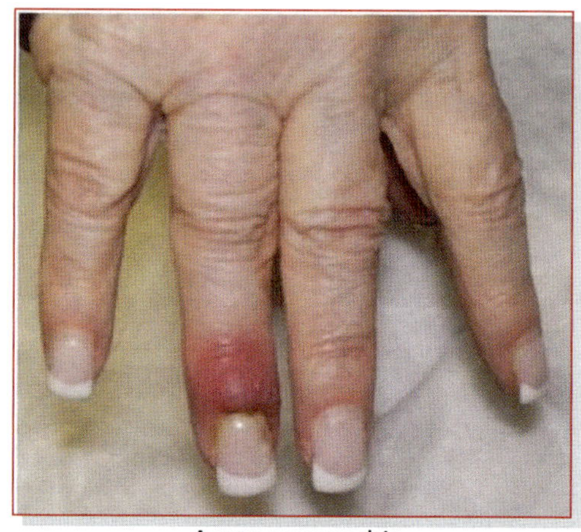
Acute paronychia

Apply a topical corticosteroid cream, such as hydrocortisone, and an antifungal cream, such as ketoconazole, for several weeks to affected nails. Avoid nail cosmetics, manicures, biting nails, and picking at cuticles while undergoing therapy. Also, limit chemical and water exposure to your nails by wearing light cotton gloves under heavy-duty vinyl gloves when performing wet work or handling chemicals. Heavy-duty vinyl gloves are available at paint stores and pharmacies. Nails can also be kept dry with nail cots, which are small rubber sleeves that fit over fingertips. They may be purchased at local and online pharmacies.

THE ACUTE FORM

Acute paronychia is a painful infection around the nail. Aggressive manicures, biting nails, and picking at cuticles may all cause acute paronychia. Bacteria can seed into the traumatized skin and cause an infection. *Staphylococci, Streptococci,* and *Pseudomonas* are the most common organisms that cause the infection.

Treatment requires draining any pus out of the infected skin. Soaking your nails in Domeboro solution for fifteen minutes three times a day will also help. Domeboro powder can be purchased without a prescription at local and online pharmacies. Finally, topical or oral antibiotics are frequently prescribed as treatment.

Pemphigus and Bullous Pemphigoid

Pemphigus (pem´fi-gŭs) and bullous pemphigoid (bul´ŭs pem´fi-goyd) are autoimmune skin diseases caused when the immune system mistakenly sends antibodies to the skin to fight an infection that does not exist. These antibodies create a split in the skin, resulting in fluid-filled bumps called blisters. Patients with pemphigus may have blistering in their mouths and on the mucosa of their private areas.

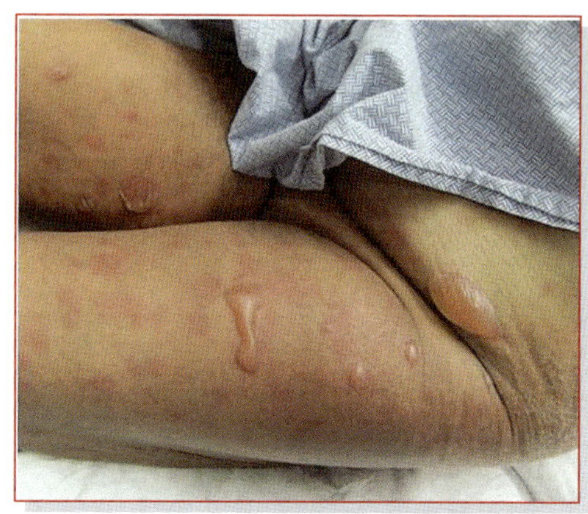

Bullous pemphigoid

Occasionally, pemphigus and bullous pemphigoid are caused by a new medicine, and if that medicine is withdrawn, the blisters may recede forever. Treatment for most other patients requires medicines that suppress the immune system. There is no definite cure for pemphigus and bullous pemphigoid, so if treatments are withdrawn, the blisters could come back.

Milder cases of bullous pemphigoid may be controlled with the daily application of a corticosteroid cream, such as clobetasol. For pemphigus and more severe cases of bullous pemphigoid, the drug of choice is usually prednisone, which is administered at relatively high doses for approximately four to eight weeks in order to get blistering under control. If new blisters continue developing after one month on prednisone, an even higher dose may be needed. If new blisters stop developing within four to eight weeks, the dose of prednisone may then be reduced. Prednisone should be taken in the early morning with food if possible, but if it causes stomach

Part I Medical Skin Conditions

upset, the daily dose can be divided into two smaller morning and evening doses.

Patients on prednisone need periodic tests to avoid side effects. For example, prednisone could cause alterations in your electrolyte levels, cholesterol levels, and blood glucose levels. Therefore, you need a fasting blood test before starting treatment. This test is repeated in one month, then every three months thereafter.

You could also develop bone degeneration during treatment, so you need a test for osteoporosis, called a DEXA scan, before starting treatment. This test is repeated every six to twelve months thereafter. You may also need vitamin D, calcium, and possibly Fosamax (alendronate) to prevent osteoporosis.

Blood pressure could also rise on prednisone, so you need a blood pressure measurement before starting treatment. This test is repeated every other month while on the medicine.

Prednisone could also cause or worsen cataracts and glaucoma, so an eye exam is needed before starting treatment. This test is repeated every six to twelve months thereafter.

Prednisone works by suppressing your immune system, thereby increasing your risk for infections. Therefore, you need a purified protein derivative skin test before starting treatment to make sure tuberculosis is not hiding anywhere in your body. Once on prednisone, if you develop an infection, call your doctor because you may need antibiotics.

Other possible side effects include stomach upset or even ulcers if taken with nonsteroidal anti-inflammatory medicines (aspirin, ibuprofen, or naprosyn), emotional agitation, suppression of the adrenal gland in long-term users, and a condition called Cushing's disease in long-term users.

The ultimate goal is to get patients on the lowest possible dose of prednisone to prevent long-term side effects. Steroid-sparing drugs help reduce your reliance on prednisone. Commonly prescribed steroid-sparing agents for pemphigus and bullous pemphigoid include dapsone, CellCept (mycophenolate mofetil), Imuran (azathioprine), methotrexate, intravenous immunoglobulin, and Rituxan (rituximab). The right drug for you will depend on the severity of your skin condition, your other medical problems, and any other drugs you take. See Part II of this book to learn about many of these steroid sparing medicines.

Pigmented Purpura

Pigmented purpura most commonly presents on the legs. The two most common types of pigmented purpura are called Schamberg's disease and Majocci's disease. Schamberg's disease is a harmless condition that appears as reddish, cayenne-pepper-colored spots. If the spots form into rings instead of spots, dermatologists call the condition Majocci's disease.

Pigmented purpura occurs when small blood vessels sitting in the skin become inflamed and burst, releasing blood into the skin. No one knows exactly what causes this, but the vessels may burst for three reasons. First, they may weaken as we age. Second, they may burst if engorged from fluid retention due to kidney failure, liver failure, heart failure, or poorly functioning valves in deep leg veins. Therefore, if you retain fluid in your legs, you may need to be checked for those conditions. Finally, drug reactions may cause the vessels to burst. Pharmaceuticals associated with pigmented purpura include carbamazepine, furosemide, glipizide, and Tylenol.

Treatment may be ineffective, and the condition may persist for years. In some patients, however, topical corticosteroid creams, such as triamcinalone or clobetasol, applied daily help significantly. Moreover, patients with leg swelling should wear compression stockings or support hose during the day to reduce swelling and alleviate the rash. The Jobst brand of support hose and compression stockings may be purchased without a prescription from surgical supply stores and local and online pharmacies.

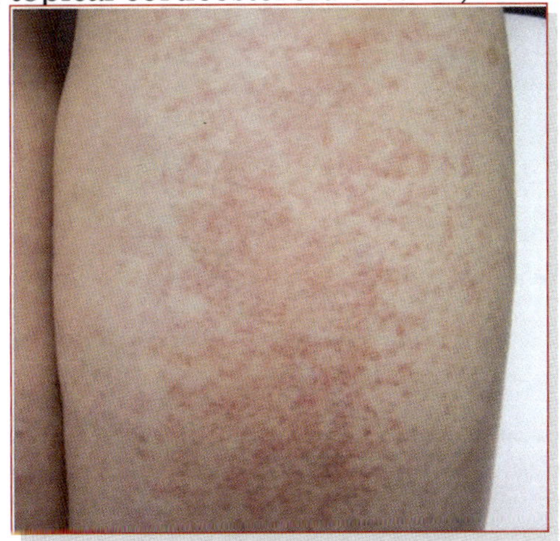

Schamberg's disease of the left leg

Pityriasis Alba

Pityriasis alba (pit-i-rī´ă-sis al´ba) is a harmless condition that presents as light-colored patches on the cheeks and neck and sometimes the arms and shoulders. It predominantly affects young people and may worsen in the summertime. No one knows what causes pityriasis alba.

Treatment begins with sun protection, and for advice on this subject please see the beginning of the essay "Skin Aging: Prevention and Treatment" in Part I of this book. Next, try applying hydrocortisone cream to the light-colored patches twice a day. Use it long enough to make the condition go away—then try moisturizing to maintain your improvement. Finally, if the condition fails to respond to a twelve-week course of hydrocortisone cream, consider a non-steroidal anti-inflammatory cream, such as Elidel (pimecrolimus cream) or Protopic (tacrolimus ointment).

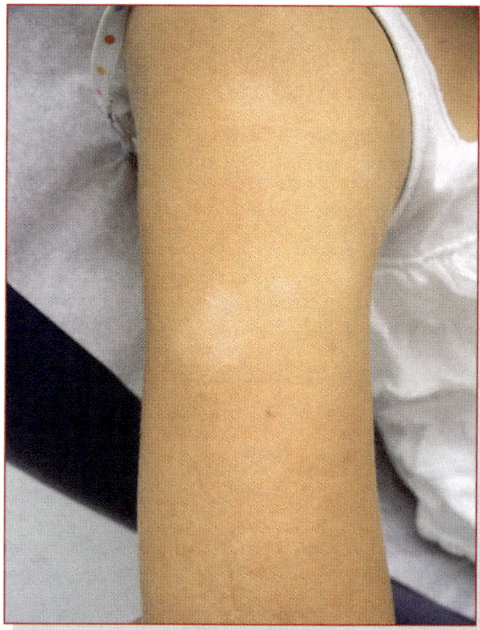

Pityriasis alba

Part I Medical Skin Conditions

Pityriasis Rosea

Pityriasis rosea (pit-i-rī´ă-sis ro´sea) is a harmless condition that resolves on its own within about six weeks. It typically starts with a single pink patch of skin that slowly enlarges. Soon thereafter, additional pink patches arise in surrounding areas. Eventually, all the pink patches fade away.

It is an autoimmune skin condition caused when the immune system mistakenly sends T cells to the skin to fight an infection that does not exist. The immune cells cause the red spots to form. What causes the immune system to malfunction in this way is unknown. In some patients, however, pityriasis rosea may result from an immune reaction to a newly started medicine. In other patients, a viral infection may cause pityriasis rosea. For example, patients often report symptoms of a viral infection, including

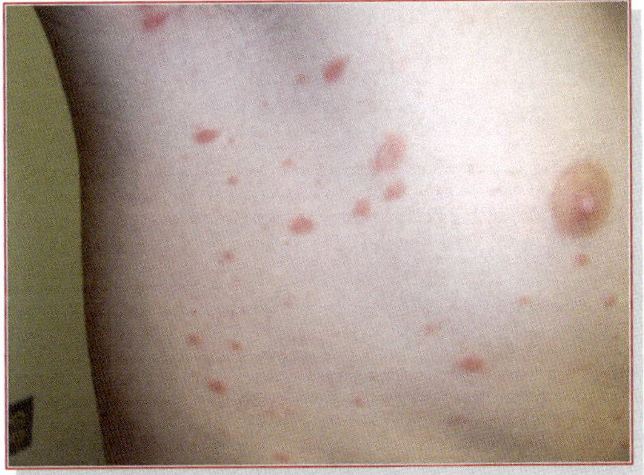

Pityriasis rosea

sore throat, cough, and runny nose. According to one hypothesis, there may be molecules in that virus that are chemically very similar to molecules found in the skin. Once the immune cells learn to recognize the virus, they identify similar molecules in the skin and travel there to fight an infection that does not exist. This inflammation causes the rash. Ultimately, the viral infection inside the body resolves, and the immune reaction in the skin resolves, too.

Apply a corticosteroid cream, such as clobetasol or triamcinalone, once daily. These creams work by removing T cells from the skin. Aveeno oatmeal baths may also soothe the skin and are available without a prescription from pharmacies. Taking 10 mg of Claritin (loratadine) in the morning and 25 to 50 mg of Benadryl (diphenhydramine) at night may also reduce itch.

Poikiloderma of Civatte

Poikiloderma (poy´ki-lō-der´mă) appears as red patches on or around the neck, chest, and arms. When it presents on the neck and chest, it is called Poikiloderma of Civatte. Upon close examination, brownish spots, reddish lines, and tiny blood vessels may be seen, and the skin texture may be slightly altered. Poikiloderma results from too much sun exposure over the course of a person's life. It does not go away, and it may spread with time. The rash may feel irritable or itchy, especially if shaved over. Creams and pills do not materially help this condition. Instead, the rash may respond to intense pulsed light treatments. See Part III of this book for more information about intense pulsed light.

Avoiding excessive sun exposure is a good idea to keep the condition from worsening. For advice on sun protection, see the beginning of the essay "Skin Aging: Prevention and Treatment" in Part I of this book.

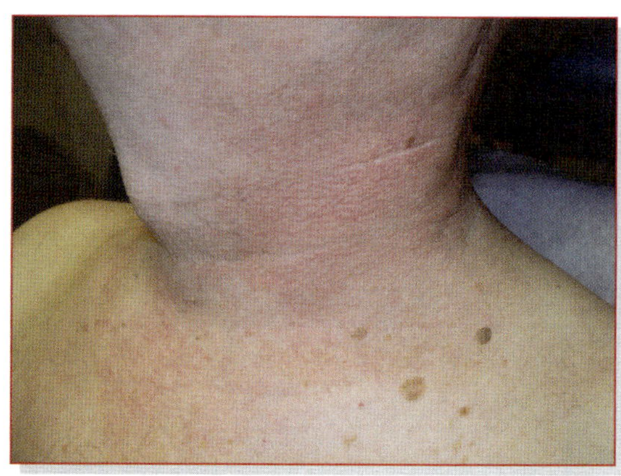

Poikiloderma of Civatte

Polymorphous Light Eruption

Polymorphous (pol-ē-mōr´fŭs) light eruption presents with itchy pink bumps that arise minutes or hours after sun exposure. Sunlight tricks the patient's immune system into sending T cells to the skin to fight an infection that does not exist. These T cells then release chemicals that cause itchy bumps that may last days or weeks. The condition often develops in the springtime and resolves by the fall.

The best treatment is prevention of excessive sun exposure. For advice on sun protection, see the beginning of the essay "Skin Aging: Prevention and Treatment" in Part I of this book. In addition, apply a corticosteroid cream, such as triamcinalone or clobetasol, to the rash daily. Narrowband ultraviolet light type B phototherapy is reserved for more persistent cases. Finally, severe cases may require prednisone or other steroid-sparing medicines, such as Imuran (azathioprine) or cyclosporine. See Part II of this book for more information about all of these treatments, which work by removing T cells from the skin.

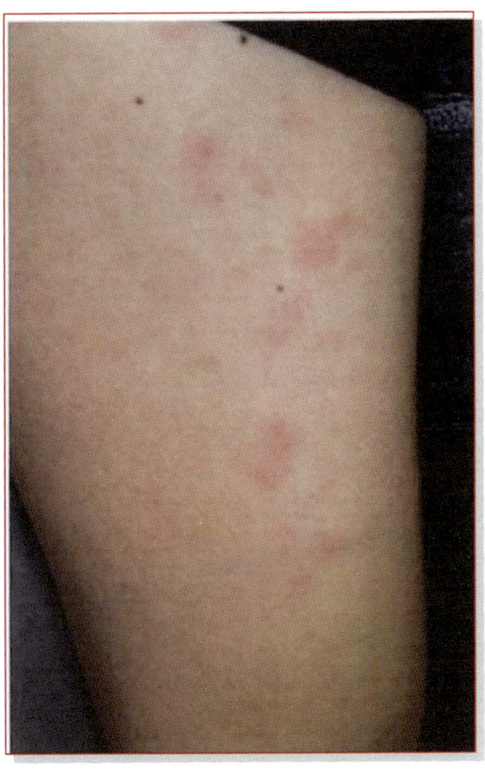

Polymorphous light eruption

Porokeratosis

Porokeratosis (pō´rō-ker-ă-tō´sis) presents as pink, skin-colored, or brown patches that appear to peel along the border. Doctors have not identified what causes porokeratosis, and there are several varieties that may arise. All variations except punctate porokeratosis can transform into skin cancer, usually appearing as a growing nodule within a long-standing skin lesion. Therefore, keep an eye on the spots. Treatments for porokeratosis include liquid nitrogen therapy, Efudex (5-fluorouracil cream), tretinoin cream, and a pill called Soriatane (acitretin).

VARIATIONS OF POROKERATOSIS

1. Linear porokeratosis arises in childhood, and lesions often have a swirled appearance.

2. Punctate porokeratosis arises around adolescence and appears as tiny bumps on the palms and soles.

3. Porokeratosis palmaris et plantaris disseminate is essentially the same condition as punctate porokeratosis, but lesions arise elsewhere on the body too.

4. Porokeratosis of Mibelli arises in childhood. Individual bumps coalesce into a large plaque, which can happen anywhere on the body.

5. Disseminated superficial actinic porokeratosis presents as scaly bumps on the arms and legs.

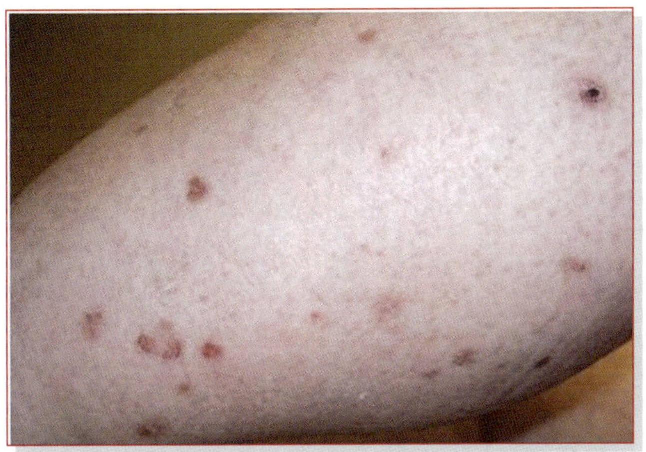

Disseminated superficial actinic porokeratosis on the leg

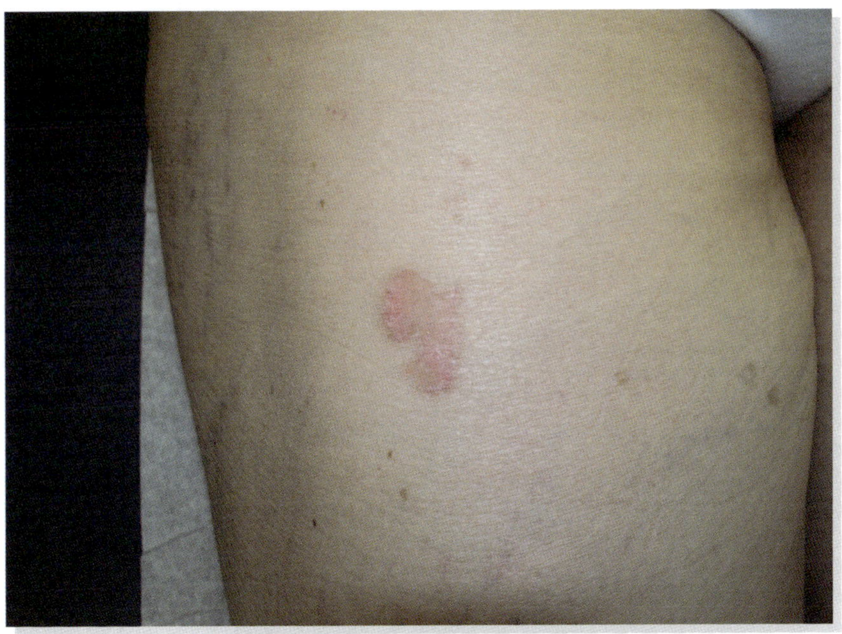

Porokeratosis of Mibelli on the thigh

Prurigo Nodularis

Prurigo nodularis (prū-rī´gō nodula´ris) presents with itchy, scar-like bumps. These bumps arise due to persistent picking and scratching. Itching is the underlying cause of prurigo nodularis, and it could result from a variety of factors, including stress, anxiety, eczema, chronic renal failure, obstructive biliary disease, Hodgkins lymphoma, polycythemia rubra vera, hyperthyroidism, gluten-sensitive bowel disease, and HIV. Your dermatologist can order tests if any of these underlying conditions is suspected.

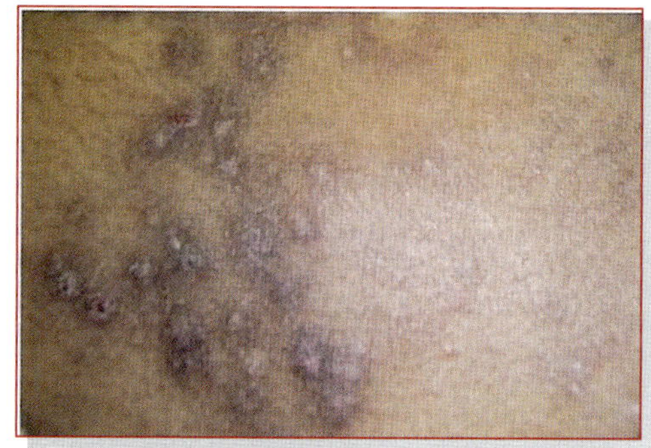

Prurigo nodularis of the upper back

Treatment requires a search for the underlying cause of itch. In addition, corticosteroid creams, including triamcinalone and clobetasol, may relieve the itch. Apply the cream once daily until the itching resolves, then stop. Restart the cream if the itch recurs. Other useful medicines include doxepin cream and capsaicin cream. Capzasin is a brand of capsaicin cream available without a prescription. Nonsedating antihistamine pills such as Allegra (fexofenadine) are often recommended for the morning, and sedating antihistamines such as Benadryl (diphenhydramine) are often prescribed for use at bedtime. Other patients may benefit from taking a low dose of a sedating antihistamine pill such as Atarax (hydroxyzine) or doxepin once or twice daily. Finally, narrowband ultraviolet light type B phototherapy and systemic immunosuppressants, such as cyclosporine and Imuran (azathioprine), are reserved for more severe cases. See Part II of this book for more information about these treatment alternatives. Finally, patients must do their best not to pick and scratch at their skin.

Part I Medical Skin Conditions

Pseudofolliculitis Barbae

Pseudofolliculitis barbae (sū´dō-fō-lik-yū-lī´tis bar´bā) is a common condition caused by tightly curled facial hair that grows back into the skin after shaving, causing severe irritation, bumps, and sometimes scars. Some people call the condition razor bumps because it presents with bumps in the beard area that arise after shaving.

There are several ways to treat pseudofolliculitis. Laser hair removal offers the possibility of a cure by eliminating the need to shave. See Part III of this book for more information about this technique. Stopping shaving and growing a beard may also cure pseudofolliculitis. If you can't grow a beard, trimming your hair

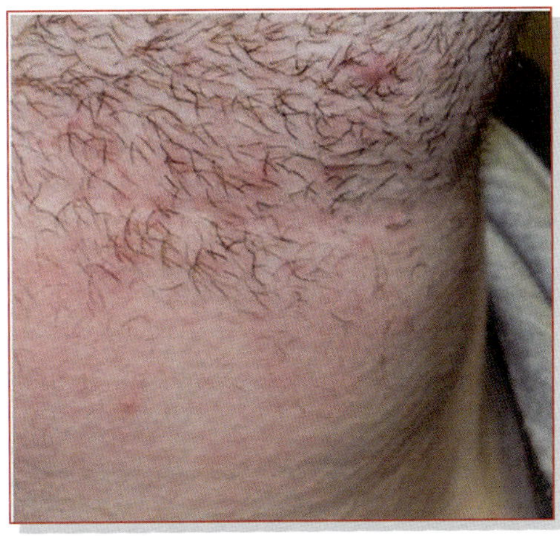

Pseudofolliculitis of the beard area

with scissors or electric clippers instead of shaving may help.

In the meanwhile, using a magnifying mirror, search for ingrown hairs daily and release them with a sterilized pair of tweezers or needle. Applying Vaniqa (eflornithine cream) twice daily to affected areas may also help by slowing the hairs' rate of growth, thus reducing the need to shave or pluck hairs. Finally, chemical depilatories, creams that dissolve hair, may improve the condition by reducing the need to shave or pluck. These creams may be purchased without a prescription.

Tretinoin cream may also help pseudofolliculitis. Apply a pea-sized drop of cream to the tip of your index finger and rub it into your fingers. Then spread a thin layer of cream onto affected skin. Applying too much cream too often may cause dryness, peeling, redness, and itching. Therefore, start by applying a small amount of cream every other night. If the cream is tolerated, after two weeks, try using it every night. If you experience dryness and peeling, try applying a smaller amount. Placing a moisturizer like Cetaphil facial moisturizer right over the cream at night and throughout the day will also reduce dryness and peeling. Finally, cutting back the frequency of cream application will alleviate any irritation. Tretinoin cream may still work if only used every third or fourth night. Finally, 1 percent hydrocortisone cream and, for severe cases, prednisone may be considered to reduce inflammation.

Psoriasis

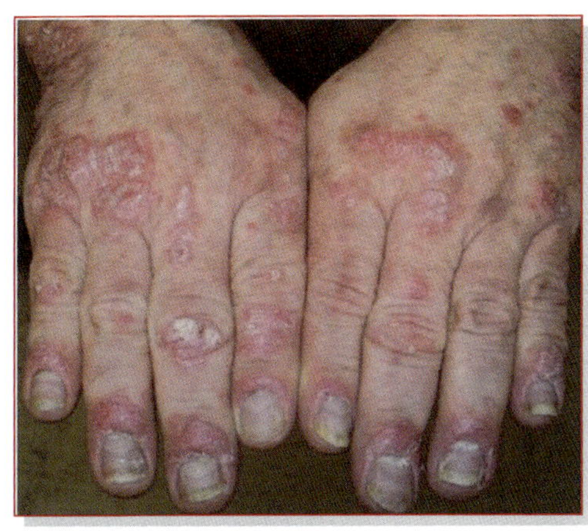

Psoriasis of the hands

Psoriasis (sō-rī´ă-sis) presents with flaky pink skin lesions. It is an autoimmune condition caused when the immune system mistakenly sends cells to the skin to fight an infection that does not exist. Once in the skin, these cells release chemicals that cause the reddish patches of skin. Psoriasis probably results from the combination of genes inherited from one's parents, since the genes are what largely program the immune system how to respond to different stimuli.

It often affects the scalp, elbows, knees, groin area, and buttock crease. If the immune cells travel to the nails, patients may develop pits and oil spots on the nails, although sometimes the nails just look yellow, resembling nail fungus. In other patients the immune cells travel to the joints, creating an inflammatory arthritis that can cause pain or stiffness of the hands, elbows, knees, hips, back, and feet. Typically, the pain or stiffness is present in the morning upon waking up, and it resolves or gets better once one gets moving. Psoriasis patients often mistakenly attribute this discomfort to old age or activities of daily living.

Many effective treatments are available for psoriasis. There are no cures, however, so if treatments are stopped, the condition could return. Topical corticosteroid creams such as triamcinalone or clobetasol are the treatment of choice for mild cases. These creams work by removing immune cells from the skin, and they work best if applied to damp skin immediately after bathing. Apply the cream daily until the rash resolves at which point the immune cells are out of the skin. Then apply a bland moisturizer, such as Vaseline or Cetaphil, to help prevent the rash from coming back. The psoriasis could recur because corticosteroid creams don't cure the problem at the genetic level. If this happens, reapply the corticosteroid cream daily until you see improvement.

Corticosteroid creams applied on a daily basis for months with no breaks can slowly start to thin out the skin. In this case, it could look shiny and wrinkled, and tiny blood vessels could appear in the skin. This side effect often resolves on its own after stopping the cream. Nevertheless, if you have used the cream daily for two weeks in a row, take a two-week break or switch to weekend use only for a while before restarting it. Moisturize your skin during the break in therapy.

Other creams that work like corticosteroid creams but will not thin out the skin include Elidel (pimecrolimus cream) and Protopic (tacrolimus ointment). However, these medicines are typically far more expensive to buy than clobetasol and triamcinalone creams, which are available in generic formulations.

Narrowband ultraviolet light type B phototherapy is the treatment of choice for more severe cases. Phototherapy works by removing immune cells from the skin. Treatments are administered in the dermatologist's office two or three times per week, and light is shined onto the skin for a few minutes for each session. The light dose is generally increased with each visit, and results are seen in approximately a month. Once the psoriasis clears, the dermatologist may stop or reduce the frequency of treatments. If your schedule does not allow you to try or continue

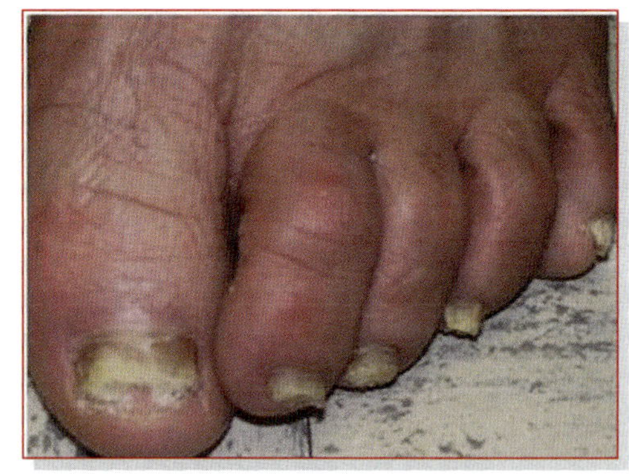

Psoriasis of the toenails.
It looks just like nail fungus.

light treatments, insurance companies may pay for an at-home phototherapy device.

Other treatments for widespread psoriasis include Soriatane (acitretin) and systemic immunosuppressants, such as methotrexate, cyclosporine, Enbrel (etanercept), Humira (adalimumab), Remicade (infliximab), and Stelara (ustekinumab). See Part II of this book for more information about these medications and narrowband ultraviolet light type B phototherapy.

Mild psoriatic arthritis is typically treated first with nonsteroidal anti-inflammatory medicines, such as naprosyn (250 to 500 mg in the morning and evening) and ibuprofen (300 to 800 mg every six to eight hours). Use the lowest dose of medicine that effectively treats the pain and stiffness. If these options do not relieve the pain adequately, other treatments including methotrexate, Enbrel (etanercept), Humira (adalimumab), Remicade (infliximab), and Stelara (ustekinumab) may be appropriate. Unlike nonsteroidal anti-inflammatory medicines, which only cover up the pain of psoriatic arthritis, etanercept, adalimumab, and infliximab may halt the destructive progression of the arthritis. Many psoriasis patients are surprised about how good their joints feel after starting these medicines.

Psoriasis is a complex condition, and patients can obtain helpful guidance by joining the National Psoriasis Foundation. Learn more about it at www.psoriasis.org.

Pyoderma Gangrenosum

Pyoderma gangrenosum (pī-ō-der´mă gangreno´sum) presents as painful open wounds. It is a type of autoimmune condition caused when the immune system mistakenly sends immune cells to the skin to fight an infection that does not exist. These cells cause pain and wound formation.

There are multiple other types of wounds that can look like pyoderma gangrenosum that must be excluded before it can be definitively diagnosed. Infections, malignancies, vasculitis, and clotting disorders can all cause open wounds that look like pyoderma gangrenosum. A biopsy of tissue from the wound border in addition to blood tests is done to help rule out these other possible causes of wounds.

There are several reasons why pyoderma gangrenosum can arise. For example, autoimmune diseases such as inflammatory bowel disease can cause it. In these cases, treatment of the underlying bowel disease may help shrink the wounds.

In other cases, pyoderma gangrenosum may arise from an underlying disorder of the bone marrow, including leukemia and monoclonal gammopathy. Blood tests, urine tests, or bone marrow tests may be needed to screen patients for these conditions. Moreover, treatment of the underlying disease may help resolve the open wounds in these patients.

Regardless of what is causing the condition, limited pyoderma gangrenosum may respond to corticosteroid injections into the open wounds. More widespread cases may require immunosuppressing drugs such as prednisone, dapsone, cyclosporine, Humira (adalimumab), and Remicade (infliximab). See Part II of this book to learn more about these medications.

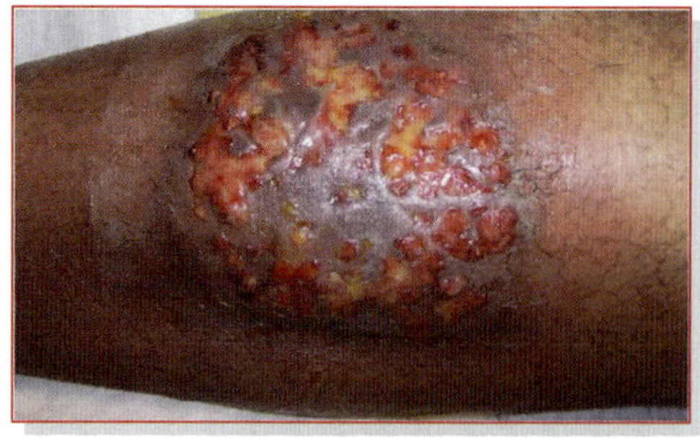

Pyoderma gangrenosum of the leg

Part I Medical Skin Conditions

Rosacea

Rosacea (rō-zāʹshē-ǎ) presents as prominent redness of the nose, forehead, mid-cheeks, and chin. Tiny blood vessels are sometimes seen in these regions, and they are the cause of the redness. Many people do not even know they have rosacea, likely because it is so common it seems normal. Others may even consider rosacea to represent prominent blushing or a normal healthy glow. In fact, rosacea has long been considered a standard of beauty; just look at the women in paintings by the French impressionist Pierre-Auguste Renoir. Most of the women in his works have rosacea, and they all look beautiful. But now it's considered a skin condition, and treatments are available for it.

Rosacea may also cause acne-like breakouts and painful lumps underneath the skin called cysts. In addition, rosacea may affect the eyes, causing a gritty sensation that sometimes feels like foreign bodies are present. Rosacea of the eyes may also cause prominent redness along the inner eyelid margins.

Some patients can identify environmental factors that trigger their rosacea. Hot beverages, alcohol, spicy foods, sun, heat, and cold are among the triggers reported. Try to identify factors that worsen your skin, and avoid them if possible. Eliminating triggers will make it easier to treat rosacea with fewer medicines.

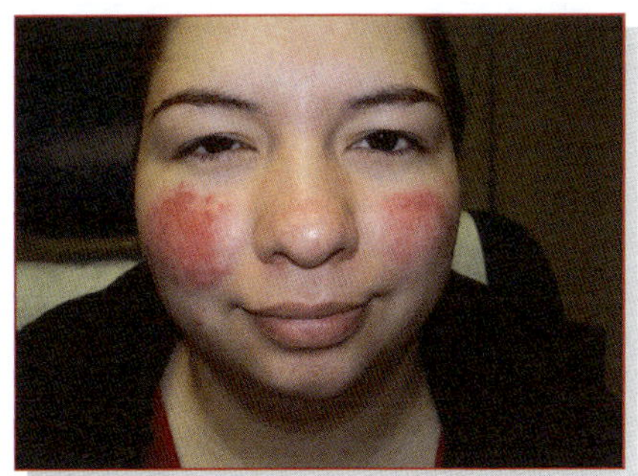

Rosacea presenting
with acne-like breakouts

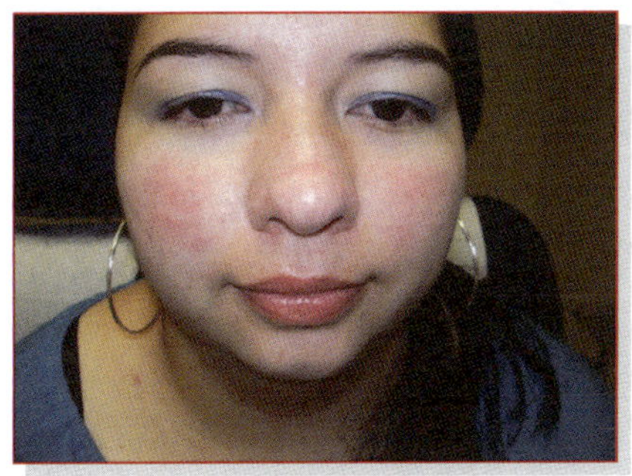

Rosacea responding
well to standard treatments

Most treatments for rosacea suppress the condition, but if stopped, the condition may return. To date, no one understands what causes rosacea, but the first-line treatments are topical antibiotic creams, gels, lotions, and washes containing the active ingredients metronidazole, sulfacetamide, sulfur, and azeleic acid. They are not designed for spot treating or for use only when getting breakouts. Instead, apply a thin layer routinely over the entire face to gradually reduce the frequency and severity of breakouts over the long term. Most treatments take a few weeks to start working, peak in efficacy after two months, and provide about 30 percent improvement. Expect slow, incremental improvement, not rapid, overnight clearance. After two months, when your medicines are fully working, go back to the dermatologist for reevaluation so he or she can make adjustments if needed. Topical treatments are also effective for rosacea of the eyes. OCuSOFT brand eyelid scrubs are available at pharmacies without a prescription.

If you need additional improvement, consider oral antibiotics, including tetracycline, doxycycline, and minocycline, which are effective for rosacea of the skin and eyes. Take them on a daily basis for maximum efficacy. Even these treatments provide only slow improvement up to a period of about two months, at which point you can expect approximately 30 percent improvement. Additional improvement is usually not seen after the two-month point. See Part II of this book for more information about oral antibiotics for rosacea. Finally, Accutane (isotretinoin) is a pill that treats the acne-like breakouts and bulbous appearing noses sometimes seen on rosacea patients. There is a chance that breakouts may never recur after a four or five month course of Accutane. Read more about this treatment option in Part II of this book.

The standard washes, creams, gels, and antibiotics for rosacea probably work better for the acne-like breakouts that are seen in rosacea than for the underlying pink skin. If the pink skin bothers you, consider undergoing intense pulsed light or pulsed dye laser treatments. These remedies utilize light of special wavelengths to target the tiny blood vessels in the skin. See Part III of this book to learn more about intense pulsed light. Dermatologists may treat larger blood vessels with electrodessication. With this technique, he or she touches the blood vessel with a device that looks like a pencil. A quick, tiny jolt of electricity from the device's tip zaps the vessel, making it disappear.

You can learn more about rosacea and how to treat it by joining the National Rosacea Society at www. rosacea.org.

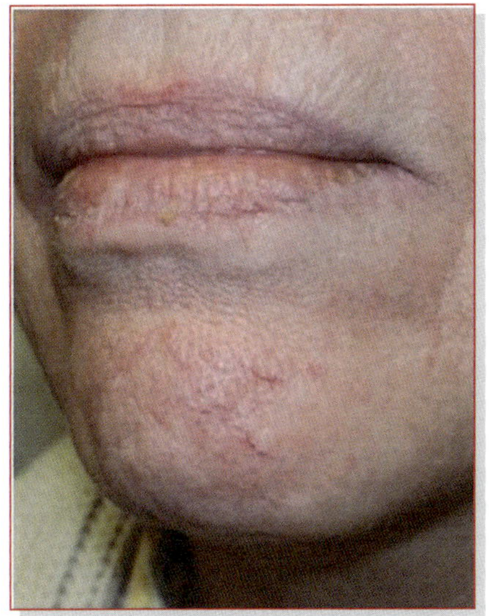

Tiny blood vessels from rosacea.

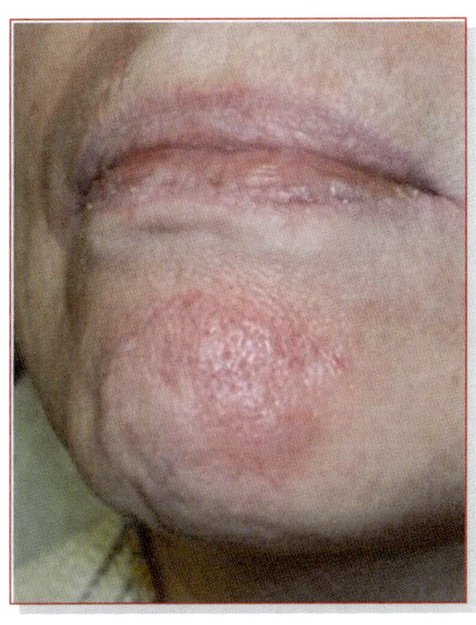

Disappearance of vessels immediately after treatment with electrodessication. Inflammation from the procedure resolves in a few hours.

Scabies

Scabies (skā´bēz) is a very itchy skin condition caused by mites that live in the skin. It is typically but not always acquired from nursing home patients, hospital patients, or groups of closely huddled people. Itching is often worse at night. A rash is often present between the fingers, on the wrists, around the nipples, in the skin folds of the stomach, around the belly button, in the groin area, or on the lower legs. The mites can leave the skin and hop onto a nearby person, so if you have scabies, all your close contacts will be at risk for contracting it.

When you first get scabies, you may not know it for a month or so. It can take that long before the itching sets in. The diagnosis may be confirmed by scraping some peeling skin from the rash and examining it under the microscope to find the mites. If a mite is seen, you have scabies. If a mite is not seen, scabies is not ruled out; mites are very difficult to find. Due to the high number of false negative results, this skin test is not always performed.

If you have scabies, you and anyone who comes into close physical contact with you needs treatment. If individuals exposed to somebody with scabies are not treated, one or more of the untreated people may contract the condition and pass the scabies mite back to everyone else. Fortunately, treatment of scabies is easy. Stromectol (ivermectin) is a

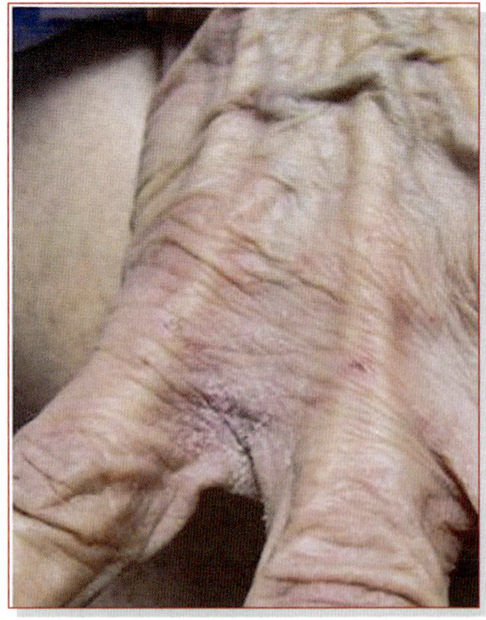

Scabies

pill you take on only two occasions: the day you pick up the prescription and fourteen days later. The first dose kills all live mites but may not kill eggs that reside in the skin. The second dose kills any baby mites that may have hatched out of eggs after the first dose was taken.

Five percent Elimite (permethrin cream) is another treatment option. You apply it on only two occasions: the day you pick up the prescription and fourteen days later. Apply it at bedtime to all skin below the neck—including all skin folds–between the toes, fingers, and in the private areas. I guarantee that mites will be hiding in any skin folds that you miss. Wash the Elimite cream off the next morning.

Mites can leave your skin and live on your clothes and linens for about three days. After that, they will die because they need rather constant contact with your skin to remain alive. Therefore, place all clothes and linens used the four days before treatment into a sealed plastic bag for four days. The mites will die there, and the clothes and linens will be safe to use again afterward.

Even after successful treatment, the dead mites remain in your skin until it completely exfoliates, which takes about one month. Therefore, an itchy rash may persist for up to six weeks after initiating therapy. During this time, itch may be treated with a corticosteroid cream called triamcinalone. If the rash abates, stop the cream and only restart it if the rash comes back. Benadryl (diphenhydramine) also helps treat itch at bedtime.

Sebaceous Hyperplasia and Fordyce Granules

Sebaceous hyperplasia (sē-bā´shŭs hī-per-plā´zē-ă) are harmless, tiny growths with a central dimple that present most frequently on the face. They arise when underlying oil glands greatly enlarge in one focal area.

The appearance of sebaceous hyperplasia can be improved with electrodessication. This technique is performed by touching the lesion with a device that looks like a pencil. A quick, tiny jolt of electricity from the device's tip zaps the spot. A tiny scab forms, which falls off in a few days. The lesion may not completely disappear afterward, but the overall appearance is usually significantly improved.

Finally, Fordyce granules are enlarged oil glands that drain onto the surface of the lips. They appear as tiny white spots. Nobody knows what causes them to form, and treatment is not available for this harmless condition.

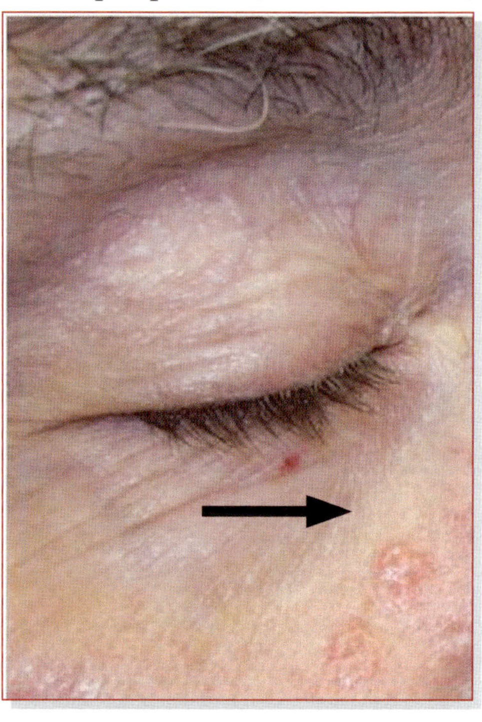

Sebaceous hyperplasia on the right cheek

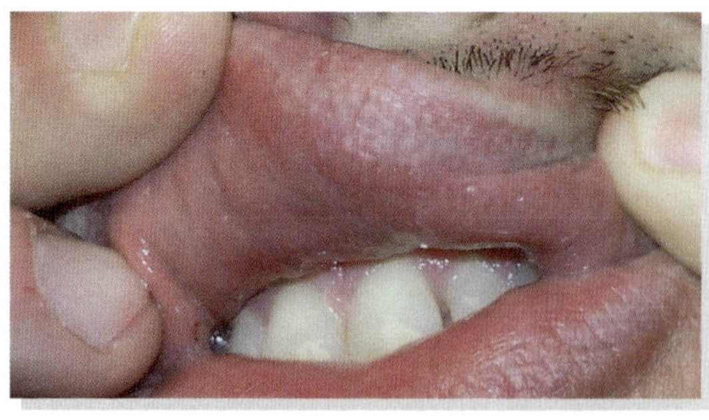

Fordyce granules on the upper lip

Part I Medical Skin Conditions

Seborrheic Dermatitis

Commonly called dandruff, seborrheic dermatitis (seb-ō-rē´-ik der-mă-tī´tis) presents on the scalp, face, ears, and sometimes chest as pinkish or skin-colored flaky patches. Occasionally these patches are very itchy. On the face, seborrheic dermatitis may arise across and between the eyebrows, around the sides of the nose, along the creases that bridge the nose to the corners of the mouth, and in and around the ears.

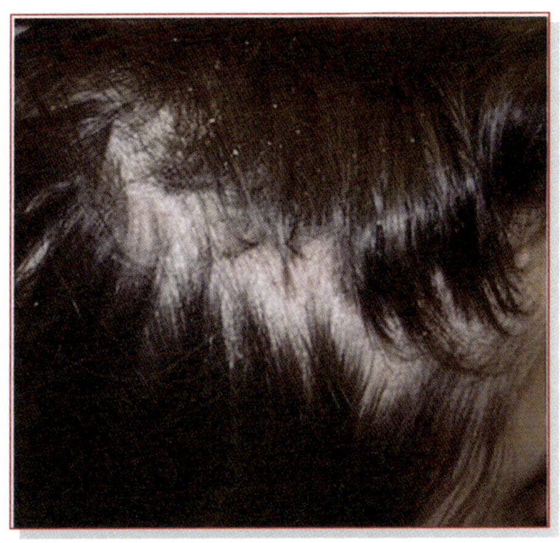
Seborrheic dermatitis

Seborrheic dermatitis may be caused by an immune reaction to a fungus that lives on the skin. Most people probably have the fungus on them because it is found all over our environment. Unfortunately, a few people develop an immune reaction to it that leads to the rash. Seborrheic dermatitis is not spread from person to person, and it is not dangerous, although it certainly can itch.

Treatments help suppress the condition, but there really is no cure, because if you stop the treatments for long enough, the rash usually recurs. Recurrences may result from the fungus finding its way back to your skin.

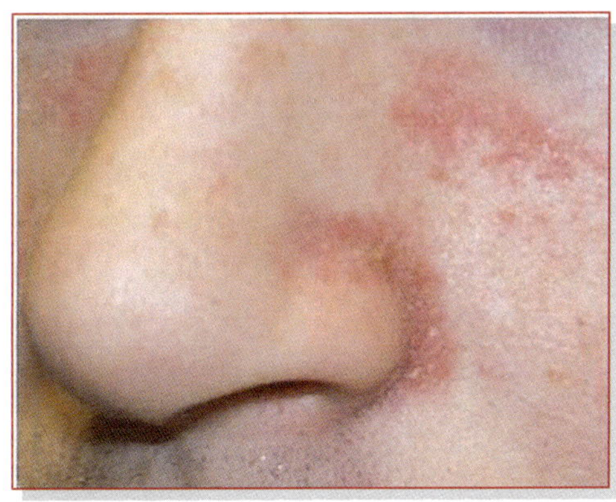
Seborrheic dermatitis of the nose and cheek

Common prescription strength treatments for the face include using 2 percent ketoconazole cream twice daily, ciclopirox olamine gel, cream or lotion twice daily, or creams, gels, lotions, and washes with 10 percent sulfacetamide with or without 5 percent sulfur twice daily. Once your skin clears up, try to find the least number of days per week needed to apply the treatment in order to maintain clear skin. On average, patients will ultimately need it every third day or every fourth day, but everyone is different.

Dermatologists treat seborrheic dermatitis of the scalp with medicated shampoos. Some are available without a prescription, including T/Sal, T/Gel, and Selsun. Other treatments are available by prescription only: 2 percent ketoconazole shampoo, Clobex (clobetasol shampoo), and Loprox (ciclopirox olamine shampoo). Lather the shampoo into your scalp for a few minutes then rinse it off. Use it as frequently as possible until the scalp clears up, and then find the least number of days per week needed to apply the treatment to maintain a clear scalp. On average, patients will ultimately need it every fourth or fifth day, but everyone is different.

Seborrheic Keratosis

Seborrheic keratoses (seb-ō-rē´-ik ker-ă-tō´sēs) are harmless growths that usually develop in adults. Doctors have not identified what causes seborrheic keratoses. They are usually tan or brown, but on the ankles they appear gray or white. Seborrheic keratoses are not cancerous, and they do not spread into the body, so they do not need to be removed. Some patients develop more of them later in life, and they can enlarge with time.

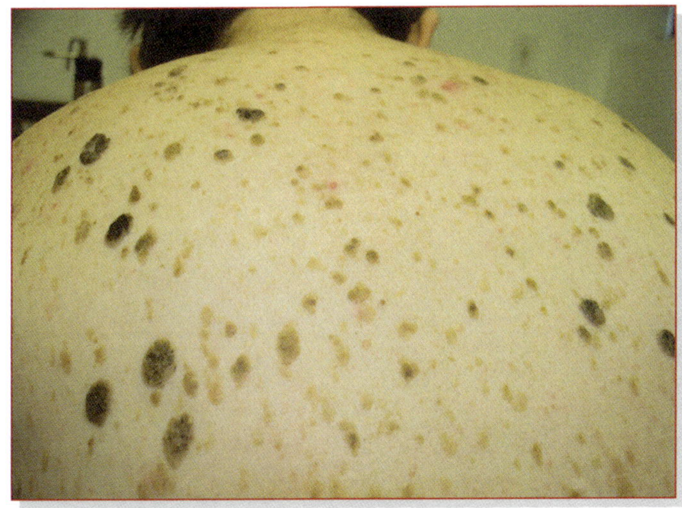

Multiple seborrheic keratoses on the back

Dermatologists commonly treat seborrheic keratoses by freezing them with liquid nitrogen. The treated growth may look like an insect bite for several hours, and within a week or two it peels off. Thus, you might want to keep your immediate social plans in mind before undergoing treatment of lesions on exposed surfaces.

Liquid nitrogen works by causing a localized frostbite on the growth, so there is a small chance a fluid-filled blister could develop in the treatment area. These freeze blisters resolve without treatment in a few days. There is also a small chance you may need a second freeze to remove the lesion. If the spot has not fallen off by one month after treatment, return for a touch-up session. No special skin care is required for the treated sites. Simply wash the sites with soap and water when bathing as you normally would.

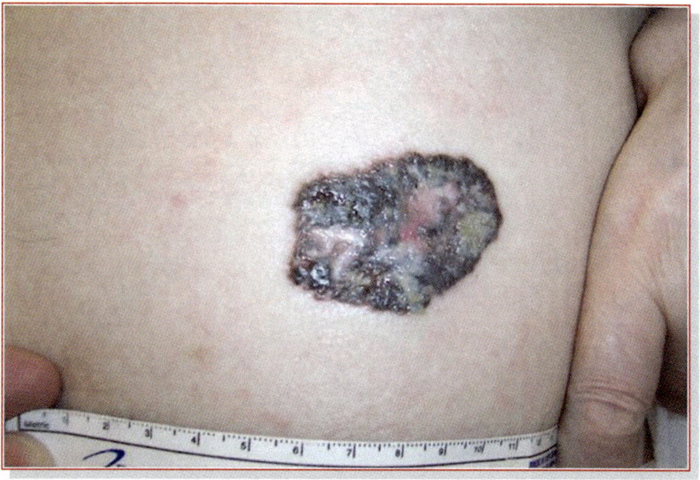

Seborrheic keratosis. Its appearance suggests the diagnosis of melanoma, but a biopsy demonstrated a seborrheic keratosis.

Shingles

Shingles (shing´glz) presents as painful or itchy fluid-filled bumps called blisters, and it usually arises in one area on one side of the body. Patients often experience a few days of pain or tingling in the area before the blisters arise. If you had chicken pox when you were younger, you can think of shingles as "return of the chicken pox." When you originally developed chicken pox, the virus traveled through the skin to your nerves, where it lay dormant for years–it never truly left your body. Then, stress or events like illnesses can trigger the virus to return to a certain area of the skin, causing blisters in a pattern called shingles. Shingles patients can spread the virus to those who've never had chicken pox, so they should avoid contact of affected skin with these people, especially pregnant women. Once all blisters have dried up, you are no longer contagious.

Once shingles starts, cover the affected skin with clothing to prevent transmission to others. New blisters may arise for one week. These blisters will dry up and form scabs within about ten days, but it can take two to three weeks before all the scabs disappear. About 10 percent of patients develop a condition called postherpetic neuralgia, which means pain at the site of the blisters. The pain may not arise until one to three months after the shingles started. It is more likely to develop in patients who experience severe discomfort before blisters arise, patients who develop very painful blisters, and patients who develop a significant number of blisters. Discomfort from postherpetic neuralgia usually resolves after several months.

Cool, wet compresses and calamine lotion help relieve itch. Applying baby powder or Domeboro soaks can also dry up blisters. Domeboro powder can be purchased without a prescription. Antiviral pills such as Valtrex (valacyclovir) are also available to reduce the extent and duration of blisters and pain. Treatment must begin within seventy-two hours of blister onset to be effective. A seven-day course is often adequate.

If your case of shingles is painful, a three-week tapering course of prednisone may reduce pain. Tylenol or nonsteroidal anti-inflammatory pain medicines such as ibuprofen and naprosyn may also help. In addition, a lidocaine patch may be applied to aching skin. Finally, gabapentin and nortriptyline are specialized pain medicines reserved for more severe cases.

Shingles is a very distressing condition that is potentially preventable. Patients age fifty and above are eligible for a vaccination that reduces the likelihood of developing shingles by boosting immunity to the chicken pox virus. Only a single vaccination is needed.

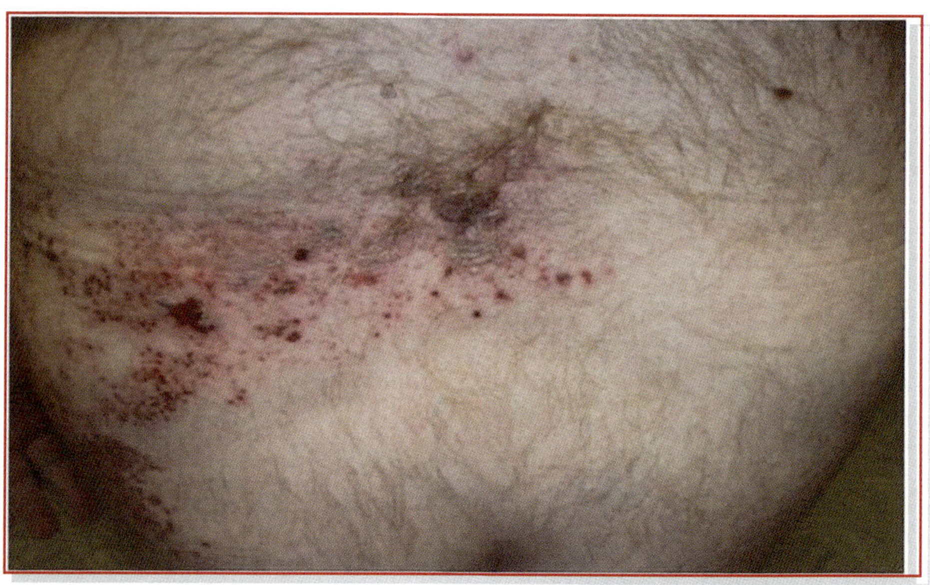

Shingles affecting the left side of the back

Part I Medical Skin Conditions

Skin Aging: Prevention and Treatment

The first step in preserving your skin's health and your youthful appearance is to avoid the harmful effects of ultraviolet light, which can cause wrinkles, moles, liver spots, rough skin patches, visible blood vessels, blackheads, and skin cancer. Therefore, avoid the intense midday sun, and schedule major outdoor activities in the morning or evening when the sun is lower in the sky.

Second, consider wearing specially designed sun-protective clothing, such as a broad-brimmed hat that protects the ears. Stylish hats and clothes designed to block the sun's harmful rays can be found at www.coolibar.com, www.sungrubbies.com, and www.sunprecautions.com.

As a third step, apply sunscreen before going outside and again every few hours while outdoors. Purchase products that block UVA and UVB light with a sun protection factor that prevents tanning and burning. Moreover, make sure the sunscreen for your face is noncomedogenic, or oil free, so it won't cause acne. Finally, patients who wear makeup should consider purchasing brands that possess sunscreen.

Avoiding too much sun, however, can lead to a deficiency in vitamin D, which may present with muscle weakness or soreness and poor balance. Therefore, report these symptoms to your doctor if they arise. Also, get plenty of vitamin D in your diet and consider a supplement if your doctor thinks this is appropriate.

ANTI-AGING TREATMENTS

In addition to preventative measures such as avoiding excessive sun exposure, there are treatments you can try to reverse signs of skin aging. Retinoid creams, such as tretinoin cream, are proven to diminish fine wrinkles and lighten liver spots and brown splotches. A few months of treatment are needed to achieve optimal results. Place a pea-sized amount of cream on your index fingertip, then rub it into your fingers, and finally apply a thin layer over your entire face, but avoid the eyelids. Apply tretinoin at nighttime because sunlight deactivates it. Using too much cream too often, however, can cause dryness and peeling. Therefore, start by applying a small amount of cream every other night. If the cream is tolerated, after two weeks, try using it every night. If this method causes dryness and peeling, try applying a smaller amount. Placing a moisturizer like Cetaphil facial moisturizer right over the tretinoin cream at night and throughout the day will also reduce dryness and peeling. Finally, cutting back the frequency of application will reduce irritation. Tretinoin cream

may still work if used every third or fourth night. Other retinoid creams are also available without a prescription, but they may not work as well.

Glycolic acid is also proven to resolve fine wrinkles and lighten liver spots and brown splotches. Best results are usually seen within a few months. If the product causes dryness and peeling, apply a moisturizer over the treated skin. Using a smaller amount on your skin or decreasing the frequency of use may also reduce irritation. DDF and Peter Thomas Roth are brands of skin care products

Part I Medical Skin Conditions

that may contain glycolic acid and can be purchased without a prescription.

Additional procedures such as superficial and medium-depth chemical peels, intense pulsed light treatments, laser resurfacing, Botox, fillers, and blepharoplasty (eyelid lift) also treat signs of skin aging. To learn more, read the essays about these procedures in Part III of this book.

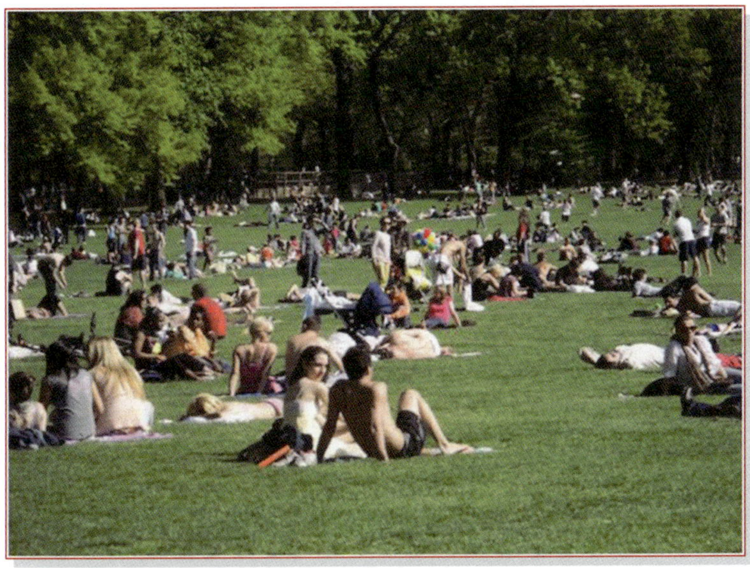

Central Park, New York City, July 21, 2010.
Everyone knows that too much sunlight can cause skin cancer, right? Sun exposure is also a prime cause of skin aging.

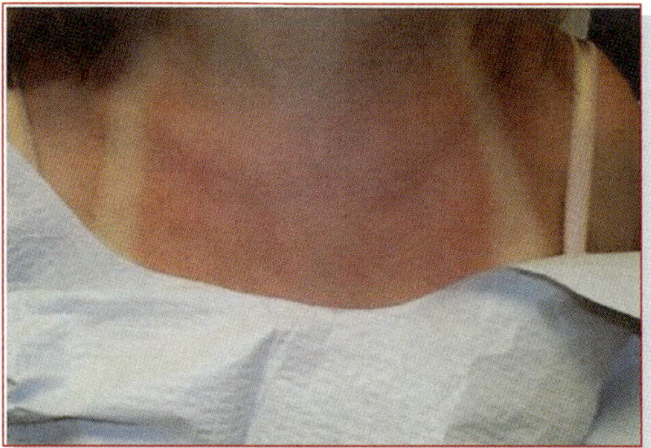

Too much sun exposure leads to a burn. A red burn and even a tan signify that damage has been done to the skin cells' DNA. Cumulative damage over the years leads to signs of skin aging and skin cancer.

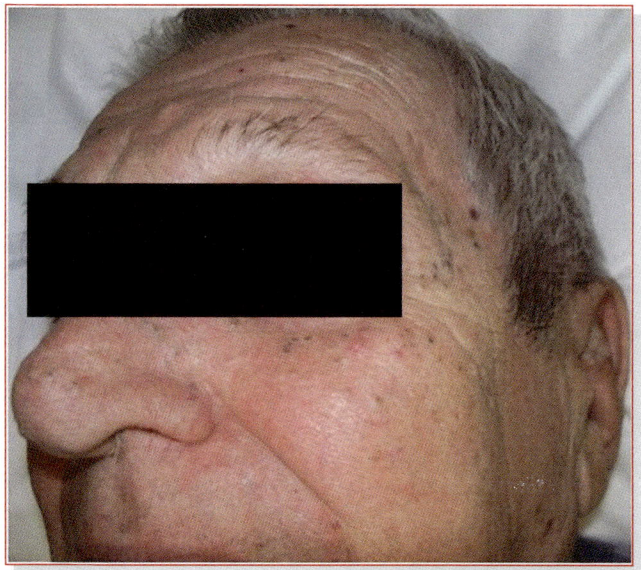

Signs of skin aging are visible including wrinkles, tiny blood vessels, and black heads. If the patient wished, the forehead lines, frown lines, and crow's feet could be treated with Botox. The blood vessels could be treated with intense pulsed light, and the blackheads could be extracted. In addition, Radiesse, Juvederm, or Restylane could make the line extending down diagonally from the corner of his nose less noticeable. He could even try laser resurfacing for any residual wrinkles. I would counsel the patient to wear a hat and sunscreen to protect his skin. Finally, he could apply tretinoin cream at night to prevent and reverse signs of skin aging.

Part I Medical Skin Conditions

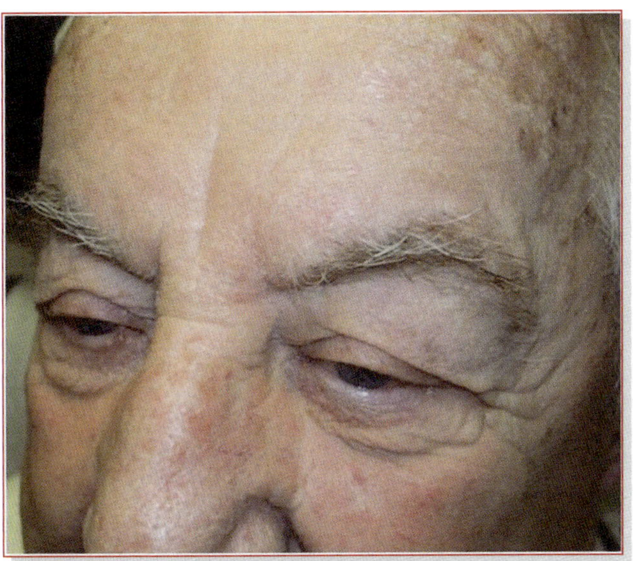

Signs of skin aging are noticeable including wrinkles, hooding of the eyelids, tiny blood vessels, and dermatoheliosis, which is a form of sun damage that makes the skin look whitish or yellowish. If the patient wished, frown lines and crow's feet could be treated with Botox, and blood vessels could be treated with intense pulsed light. Dermatoheliosis could be treated with laser resurfacing, and hooded eyelids could be treated with blepharoplasty. To protect his skin against future aging, the patient should wear a hat outside and apply sunscreen daily. He could also apply tretinoin cream at night to prevent and reverse signs of skin aging.

Skin Tag

Skin tags are very common soft, skin-colored growths that tend to arise on the neck, armpits, and eyelids. Nobody knows what causes them or how to prevent more from arising in the future. Skin tags may stay the same size, but they could get bigger. If they get scratched off, they may bleed.

Skin tags are harmless and may be left alone. However, very irritating skin tags are easily treated. Dermatologists remove them without anesthesia, using surgical scissors. The doctor may, however, inject lidocaine into very large skin tags before removal to reduce discomfort. Once removed, skin tags do not grow back.

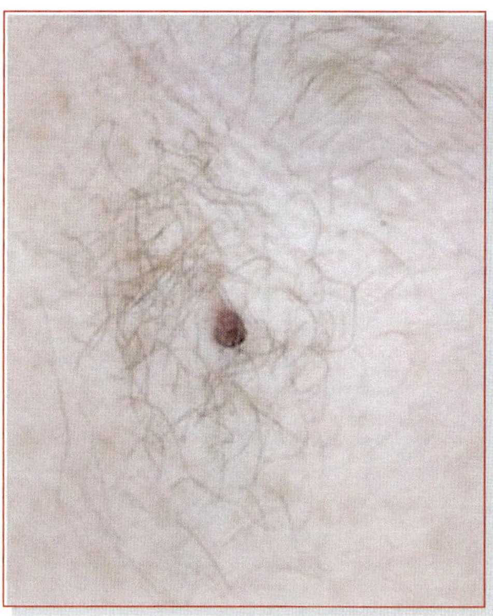

Skin tag of the left armpit

Squamous Cell Carcinoma

Squamous cell carcinoma (skwā´mŭs sel kar-si-nō´mă) is the second-most common type of skin cancer. It usually presents as a pinkish growth with a rough, raised surface. Squamous cell carcinoma is caused by the harmful effects of sunlight over many years or decades. Sunlight damages the DNA in skin cells to the point where the cells proliferate abnormally.

Without treatment, a squamous cell carcinoma slowly grows to cover more area. Once this starts happening, there is a small but real chance that the cancer could spread to the rest of the body. Fortunately, this is very unlikely to happen if the growth is treated while it is still small.

A variety of treatments are available for a squamous cell carcinoma. If the growth is superficial and has not started to grow deeply into the skin, and it is not located on the face, the dermatologist may treat it with a cream called Aldara (imiquimod).The patient applies the cream to the growth and a small area of normal-looking skin around it at night, and then rinses it off in the morning. Applications are repeated five nights per week, usually Monday through Friday, for approximately six weeks. The area becomes very red and crusty during treatment, and patients should consider this cosmetic issue before proceeding with this

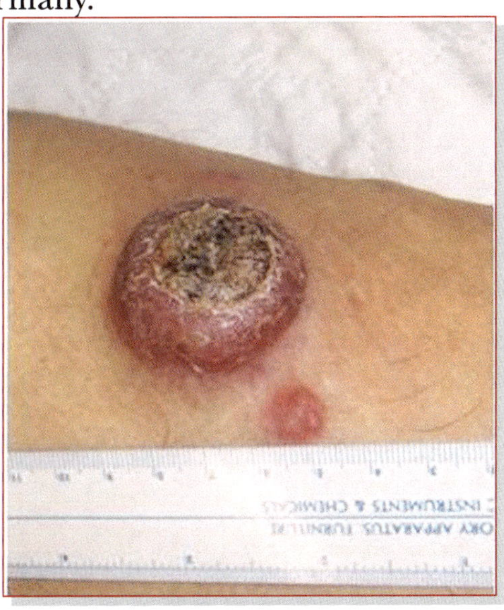

Squamous cell carcinoma

technique. Moreover, stop the cream and consult your doctor if you develop significant discomfort at the treatment site. Finally, Efudex (5-fluorouracil cream) applied twice daily for up to six weeks works in a manner similar to Aldara.

The dermatologist may also treat superficial squamous cell carcinomas with a technique called electrodessication and curettage. With this technique, the doctor first injects lidocaine into the growth to numb the area. He or she then uses an instrument that makes the cancer form a scab, which is scraped away painlessly. This procedure takes about fifteen minutes.

A third method of treating superficial squamous cell carcinomas uses liquid nitrogen, which the dermatologist sprays onto the spot, causing a localized frostbite on the growth. The skin cancer forms a scab within about two weeks and then falls off. This procedure

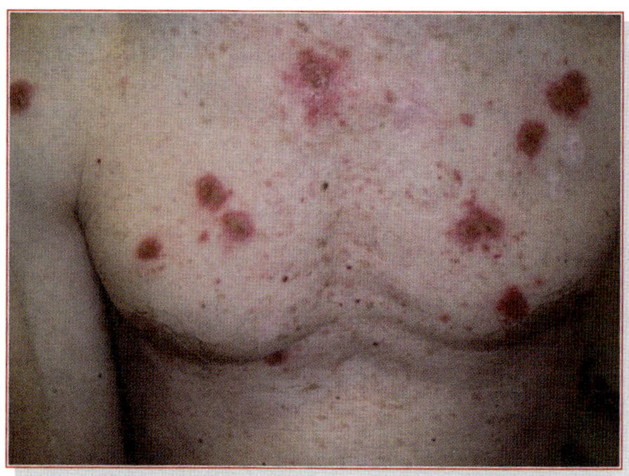

Multiple superficial squamous cell carcinomas undergoing treatment with Efudex cream

takes about one minute in the dermatologist's office. The disadvantage of liquid nitrogen, electrodessication and curettage, and Aldara and Efudex creams is that patients never receive confirmation from a pathologist that the cancer is all out.

If the cancer has spread deeply into the skin, the dermatologist is likely to recommend excising the growth. He or she first injects lidocaine around the lesion to numb the area. The doctor then removes more tissue around the spot in a painless manner with a scalpel. Finally, sutures are placed to close the surgical site. The entire process requires one hour. Afterward, the specimen is submitted to a pathologist to confirm it was completely removed, and

Part I Medical Skin Conditions

patients return in two weeks for suture removal. Excisions are also reasonable for superficial squamous cell carcinomas because they confirm the cancer is completely out. Read more about excisions in Part IV of this book.

Finally, if the skin cancer is very large or is on the face, Mohs micrographic surgery should be considered. Mohs surgeons are dermatologists with special training who perform this procedure in the office. The surgeon first injects lidocaine into the growth to numb the area. He or she then removes the cancer and a small moat of normal looking skin around it with a scalpel. The same doctor then examines the specimen under the microscope while you wait in the office to confirm that it has been removed completely. Once it's all out, the surgeon repairs the site. This surgical method is discussed in greater detail in Part IV of this book.

Patients with squamous cell carcinoma are at risk for developing additional skin cancers and need a full skin examination to make sure the rest of their skin is normal. Patients should also limit their sun exposure to help prevent the development of additional skin cancers in the future. For advice on sun protection, see the beginning of the essay "Skin Aging: Prevention and Treatment" in Part I of this book.

Stasis Dermatitis

Stasis dermatitis (stā´sis der-mă-tī´tis) can arise abruptly as an itchy, pink rash on the legs. This presentation is called acute stasis dermatitis. However, when stasis dermatitis persists for years, it can leave non-itchy rust-colored patches on the legs and is called chronic stasis dermatitis. Finally, if stasis dermatitis is severe enough, a patient can develop open wounds called stasis ulcers.

Stasis dermatitis typically develops in adulthood when leg veins stop working as well, and blood in the legs has trouble returning to the heart. Fluid retention in the legs may also result from kidney failure, heart failure, liver failure, and as a side effect of medications. Visible bulging veins may arise on the legs, and the stagnating blood releases chemicals into the skin that cause the rash. Many patients will also complain of swelling and leg aches, particularly after standing all day. Fewer patients will have restless legs at night.

Topical corticosteroid creams, including triamcinalone or clobetasol, are the first-line treatment. Apply the cream daily until the itching, redness, and flaking reside. At this point stop the cream, but restart the cream if the rash recurs. If you use topical corticosteroids daily for two weeks in a row, take a two-week break or switch to weekend use only for a while to allow the skin to recover. Even after successful treatment, some rust-colored or purplish color may persist, and creams do not remove this pigment.

Other treatments are important for controlling stasis dermatitis. For example, raise your legs on a table, ottoman, or recliner when sitting to help return blood in the legs to the heart. This intervention alone may alleviate the rash and pare the amount of topical corticosteroid cream needed. Wearing support hose or compression stockings during the day is also important. They compress leg veins and help return blood in the legs back to the heart. Potential benefits include less leg aching, mitigation of the rash, and a reduction in the amount of topical corticosteroid cream needed. The Jobst brand of support hose and compression stockings may be purchased without a prescription at pharmacies and surgical supply stores.

If your legs develop open wounds, special dressings called Unna boots may be recommended by your dermatologist (see top figure on page 129). A moist, zinc-coated wrap is applied to your foot and leg. Then a dry elastic wrap secures the first dressing in place. Unna boots are typically left on for several days, after which they are changed. Wounds may require several weeks to heal in this manner.

If stasis dermatitis does not respond well to treatment, your medical doctor may need to examine and treat you for possible causes of fluid retention, including kidney, heart, and liver failure. In addition, medications that can cause leg swelling may need to be stopped. Finally, your deep leg veins may need evaluation with a duplex Doppler ultrasound, which can be done at the radiology department of many hospitals. If defective veins are found, the doctor may remove them or treat them with a laser. These interventions can potentially alleviate leg aches, rash, and open wounds.

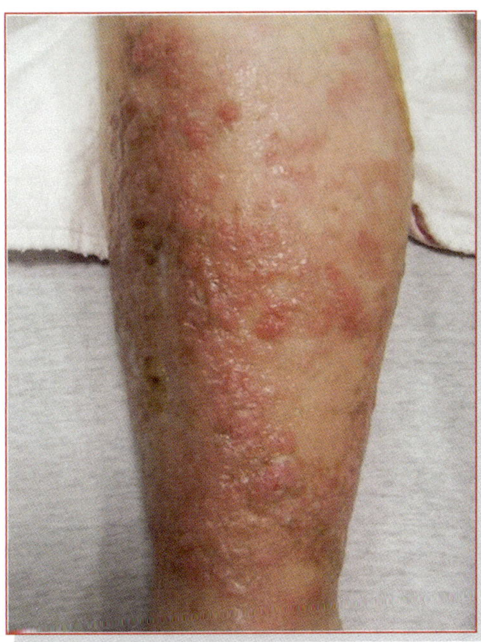

Acute stasis dermatitis. Notice the large volume of fluid trapped in the skin.

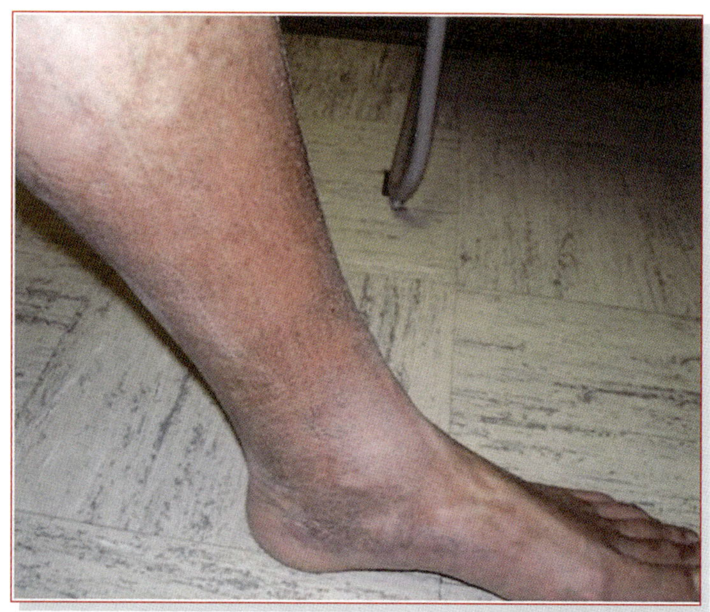

Chronic stasis dermatitis.

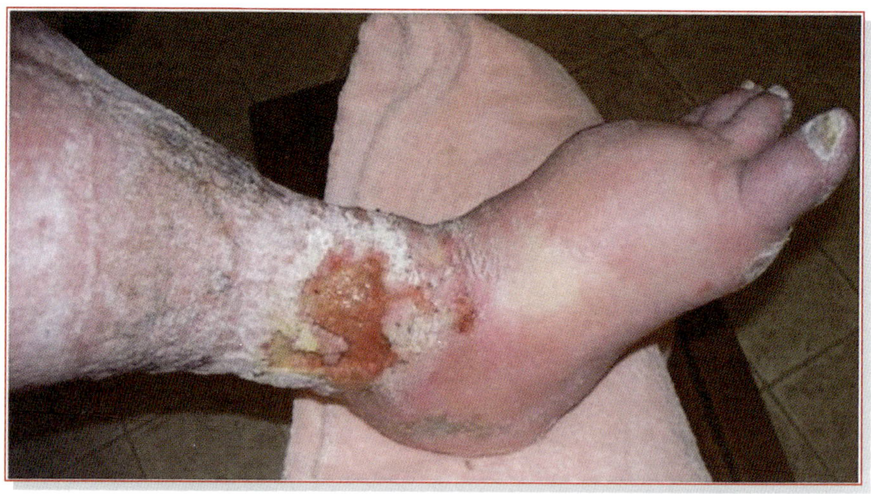

Stasis ulcer resulting from severe swelling in the lower leg. White triamcinalone cream was applied to the surrounding stasis dermatitis.

Part I Medical Skin Conditions

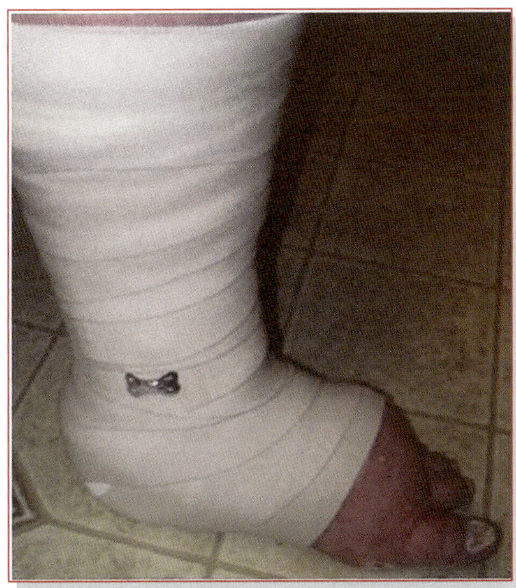

Unna boot applied to the patient shown on the bottom of the opposite page.

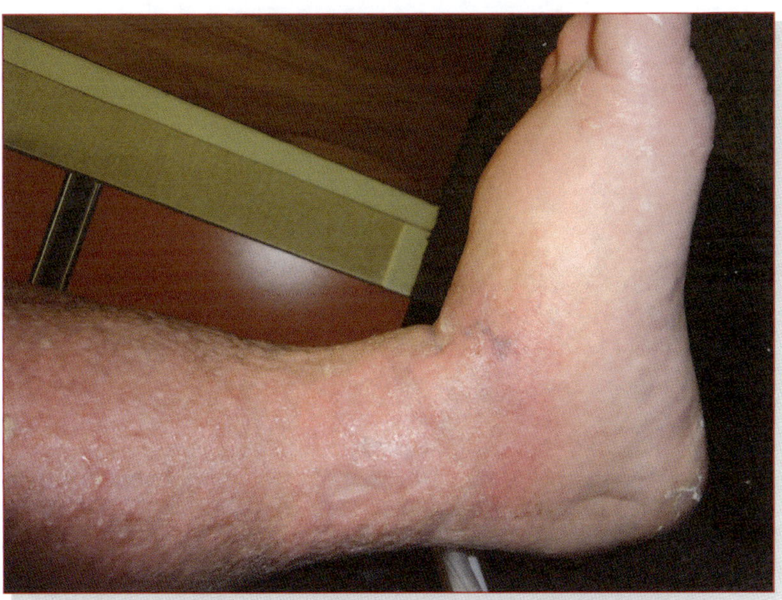

Stasis ulcer healed after repeated application of Unna boots.

Telogen Effluvium (Hair Loss)

Telogen effluvium (tel´ō-jen e-flū´vē-ŭm) is a common cause of hair loss. Patients typically notice shedding of hair into the sink or on the hairbrush. It is normal to lose between fifty and one hundred hairs per day, but when shedding significantly exceeds this amount, telogen effluvium should be considered.

Telogen effluvium may result from a very stressful event such as a surgery, illness, death in the family, relationship issue, money problem, or legal issue. Other common causes include new medicines and iron or thyroid hormone deficiency. Medicines more commonly associated with telogen effluvium include hormone replacement therapy, nonsteroidal anti-inflammatory medicines for pain, anticoagulants, beta blockers for high blood pressure, and drugs for high cholesterol.

Hair loss typically follows the inciting event by several weeks and may last for half a year or more. Telogen effluvium may lead to a decline in hair density over the scalp, but it does not lead to total hair loss. Eventually, the hair regrows. Treatment may include Rogaine (minoxidil) applied twice daily for months. It works by stimulating hair growth. Rogaine is available in solution and foam formulations, and it comes in 2 and 5 percent concentrations. The more expensive foam formulation tends to absorb better into the scalp, while the solution formulation may drip down onto the cheeks, where it could grow hair. Patients who attain good results with minoxidil should discontinue it with some caution, because if stopped for long enough, they may gradually lose the progress they have achieved. Finally, many pregnant women report enhanced hair growth while on prenatal vitamins, so this intervention may also be worth a try.

Tinea Versicolor

Tinea versicolor (tin´ē-ă versic´olor) is a whitish, brownish, or pinkish rash that usually presents on the chest, back, or shoulders. Sometimes the rash is covered with a fine scale. The rash is caused by a fungus called *Malassezia globosa* or *Malassezia furfur* that lives on human skin and eats skin oils. It is hard to tell where exactly a patient may have acquired the fungus because it is present everywhere. Fortunately, the rash is not serious and is easily treated.

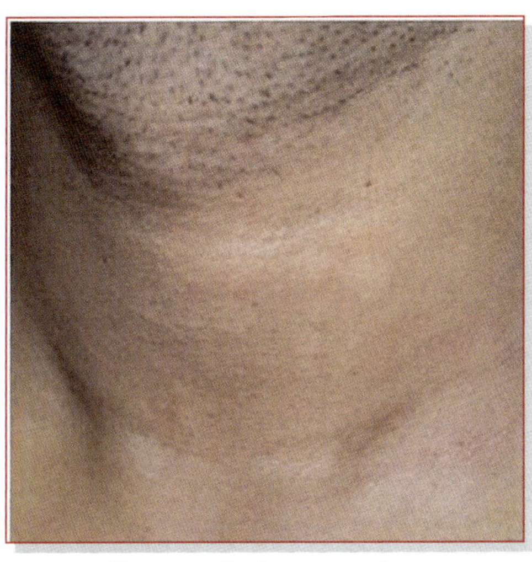

Tinea versicolor presenting as light, tan-colored patches

Patients desiring topical therapy may apply 2.5 percent selenium sulfide lotion to the rash for ten minutes then rinse it off. Treatments should be performed daily for one week. To prevent the rash from recurring, consider repeating the weeklong application routine once a month for three months.

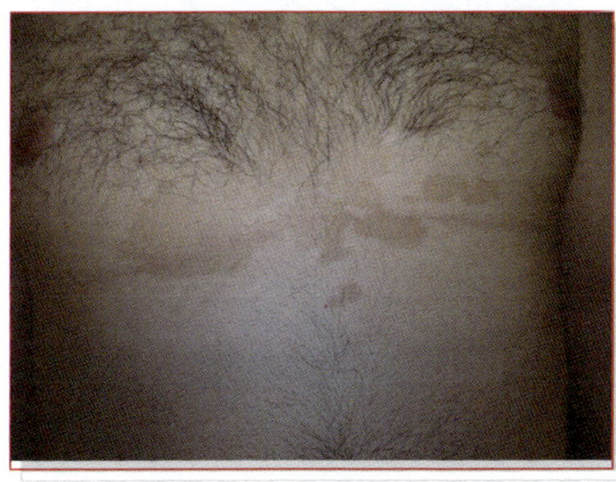

Tinea versicolor appearing as brown patches on the chest

Tinea versicolor also responds to ketoconazole pills. After taking two tablets, exercise to the point of sweating—this helps get the medicine into your skin. One week later, take another two tablets in the same fashion. Finally, consider repeating this ritual once a month to prevent recurrences.

Vitiligo

Vitiligo (vit-i-lī´gō) presents with loss of skin pigmentation in focal patches. The skin appears chalk white when exposed to a special lantern called a Woods lamp. Doctors are still researching the cause of vitiligo, but they believe it may be an autoimmune disease caused when the immune system mistakenly sends T cells to the skin to fight an infection that does not exist. These T cells may kill the pigment producing cells in the skin. The course of vitiligo is unpredictable. In some people it does not progress, but it can become widespread in others. Finally, some patients may develop other genetically related autoimmune conditions such as thyroid disease, diabetes, and pernicious anemia. Patients demonstrating obvious signs of these conditions should be tested for them.

Topical corticosteroid creams, such as clobetasol and triamcinalone, are the treatment of choice for limited vitiligo. They may work by removing T cells from the skin. Apply them once or twice daily, and a few months are needed to see results. Corticosteroid creams applied daily for months with no breaks can slowly start to thin out the skin, resulting in a shiny and wrinkled look, and tiny blood vessels could appear in the skin. This side effect often resolves on its own after stopping use of the cream. Nevertheless, if you have used the cream daily for two weeks in a row, take a two-week break or switch to weekend use only for a while before restarting it.

Other creams that work like corticosteroid creams but will not thin out the skin include Elidel (pimecrolimus cream) and Protopic (tacrolimus ointment). Elidel and Protopic are typically far more expensive to buy than clobetasol and triamcinalone creams, which are available in generic formulations.

More widespread vitiligo is more practically treated with narrowband ultraviolet light type B phototherapy. This modality may work by removing T cells from the skin. Treatments are administered two or three times a week for at least two months. Once repigmentation of the skin occurs, treatments may be stopped or tapered off.

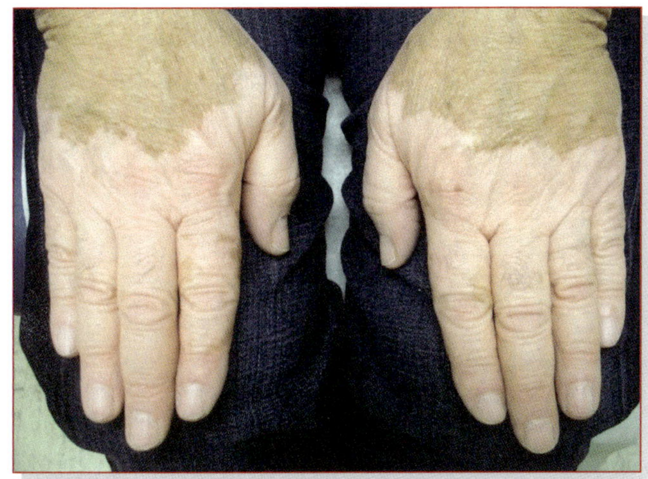

Vitiligo

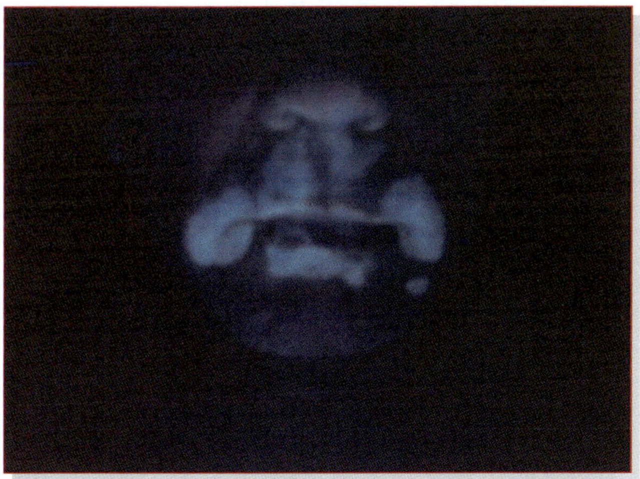

Chalk white appearance of vitiligo when exposed to a Woods lamp

Wart

Warts are caused by a virus that finds its way into the skin and causes skin cells to proliferate until a growth forms. Patients may inadvertently acquire the virus by contact with someone else who has a wart. Warts can also be transmitted by scratching one location, which picks up the virus under the fingernails, and then scratching somewhere else and depositing the virus there. If left alone, warts may resolve on their own. However, they may persist for years and spread if not treated.

Most warts require a few treatments on a monthly basis to resolve, so be patient. The most common treatment is liquid nitrogen, which, when sprayed onto a wart, causes a localized frostbite. The dermatologist may then apply monochloroacetic acid on the wart, which kills the cells that harbor the wart virus. The acid is covered by a small adhesive bandage and rinsed off the next morning. If you develop any tenderness at the site of acid application, remove the bandage and wash the area with water. After treatment, the wart should peel off within a week or two. Keep in mind that the freezing effect of liquid nitrogen could cause a fluid-filled bump to form in the area. These freeze blisters always resolve on their own without treatment. Finally, return to the dermatologist in one month to treat any wart roots that may remain in the skin. If not removed promptly, these roots may regenerate the original wart.

Another effective treatment for warts is immunotherapy with *Candida* yeast and *Trichophyton* fungi. The dermatologist injects mashed

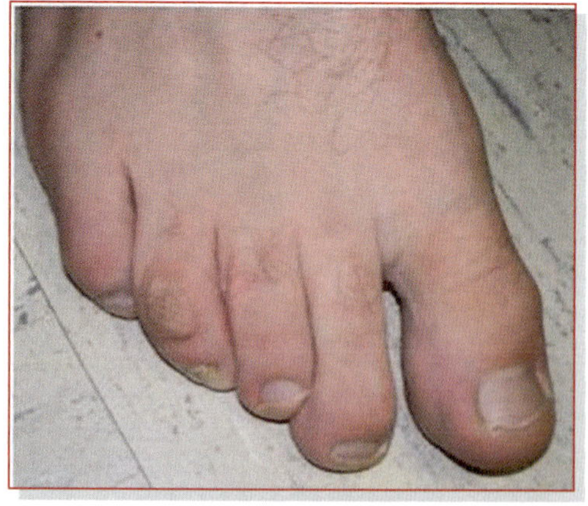

Wart of the right fourth toe

Part I Medical Skin Conditions

up, killed forms of *Candida* and *Trichophyton* into the warts to stimulate immune cells to come into the area, where they learn to recognize and kill the wart virus. A few monthly injections are often needed to clear warts.

Aldara (imiquimod) cream is also used to treat warts. Apply a small dab of cream to the warts at bedtime, and cover them with a small adhesive bandage. Then, fold up the medicine packet and save any unused cream in the refrigerator for use the next night. Wash off the cream in the morning, and repeat this procedure five to seven times a week for a few months. Imiquimod stimulates your immune system to attack the virus that causes warts. For this reason, treated warts may look red and inflamed—that is expected and may signify that the treatment is working. If you develop discomfort at the treatment site, stop the cream for a while and consider starting application again but less frequently after the discomfort subsides.

Tagamet (cimetidine) is another treatment for warts that may work by stimulating the immune system to attack the wart virus. Cimetidine is a pill prescribed according to a patient's weight (20 to 40 mg/kg/day), and it is usually taken for up to three months. The most common side effect is stomach upset.

Other home-based therapies are available from pharmacies without a prescription. Using them may add to the effectiveness of office-based treatments such as liquid nitrogen. Home-based therapies are typically started one week after the wart was treated in the office. If the product's active ingredient is salicylic acid, use it until the wart turns white, and then peel the dead skin off.

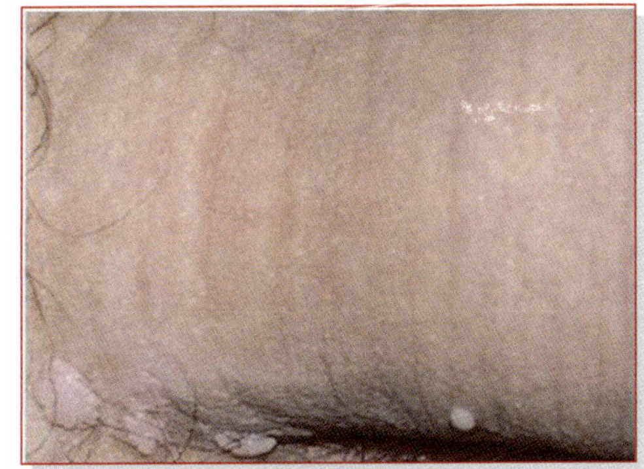

Genital warts

Continue using the home-based therapy as much as possible until your next office visit.

Warts presenting on private parts are considered genital warts and are sexually transmitted. The virus in genital warts may sometimes lead to cancer in both women and men. The consistent use of condoms helps prevent the spread of warts and the virus to one's partner. Vaccinations (Gardasil) are also available for patients nine to twenty-six years of age to prevent the acquisition of genital warts. Three vaccinations are required on a monthly basis for optimal results.

Part II
Medical Treatments

Accutane (Isotretinoin)

Isotretinoin is an appropriate treatment for severe acne and rosacea that presents with painful lumps under the skin and scarring. Isotretinoin is by far the strongest treatment for these conditions and can even lead to a cure. Other types of treatments will suppress acne and rosacea but cannot lead to a cure. Typically, dermatologists have patients try the strongest topical creams and washes and oral antibiotics for a few months before isotretinoin is considered.

Isotretinoin is a heavily regulated drug because it can cause birth defects in children born to women on the drug. For this reason, sexually active women must use two forms of contraception for one month before the drug is started and until one month after the drug is discontinued. In addition, they need to have two pregnancy tests with negative results before starting treatment and one per month during treatment.

Dry eyes, lips, and skin are the most common side effects seen with isotretinoin. Wearing contact lenses is not safe if one's eyes dry out. Artificial tears may even be needed to hydrate the eyes. In addition, patients who develop dry lips should use Aquaphor, an ointment available without a prescription. Finally, apply a moisturizer to treat dry skin. Moisturizers work best if applied to damp skin after bathing. A variety of products are suitable, including Cetaphil and CeraVe, but there is no best option. The one that feels best on your

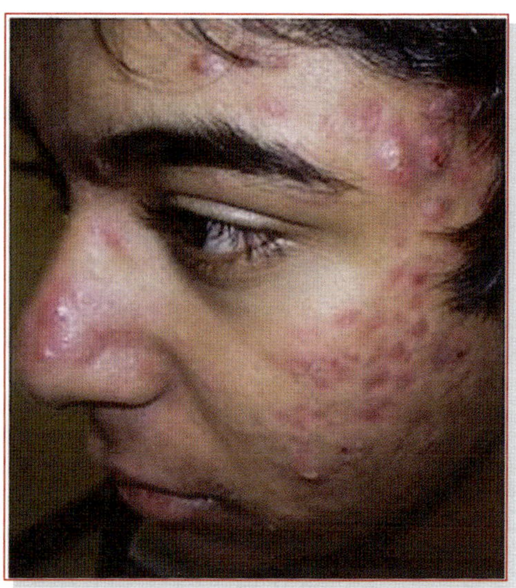

Severe acne

skin may be different than the one that feels best on someone else's skin.

Periodic blood tests are also needed to help avoid side effects. For example, isotretinoin can raise cholesterol levels, in rare cases high enough to inflame the pancreas. Isotretinoin can also cause liver inflammation in rare cases. Finally, blood cell counts could drop during treatment. For all these reasons, a fasting blood test is needed before starting treatment, and this test is repeated monthly during therapy.

Mood changes are another possible effect of isotretinoin, and there are rare reports of depression and even suicide during treatment. However, it is unclear if isotretinoin caused these events, which must be very uncommon, because patients routinely become much happier on the medicine as they watch their skin clear up. Finally, there are rare reports of ulcerative colitis, an intestinal disease, developing after starting the medicine. Again, it is uncertain if isotretinoin caused these cases, which may have arisen in these patients even if they had never started the medication.

Isotretinoin is dosed according to the patient's weight. The target dose is one mg/kg/day, but I usually start patients on half that dose for the first month to help them tolerate it. The cumulative dose at the end of about five months is usually 120 to 150 mg/kg.

Before starting isotretinoin, patients must learn about treatment guidelines enforced by iPLEDGE, a program that

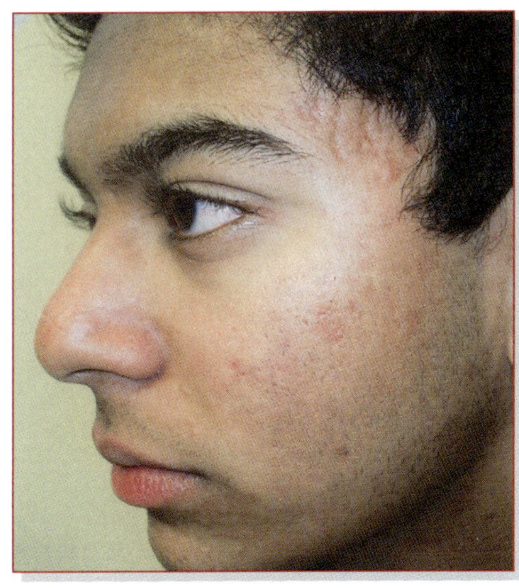

Improvement from isotretinoin. The dermatologist could treat the residual scars with laser resurfacing.

regulates how doctors can prescribe the medicine. This program was established to prevent pregnancies in female patients on the medicine, but male patients are also subject to the regulations. Learn more about the program at www.ipledgeprogram.com. Dermatologists will provide interested patients with an iPLEDGE booklet, which must be read, signed, and returned to the doctor's office before a prescription can be written. Women should pay particular attention to what kind of contraception they will need and when they should get their pregnancy tests. Finally, physicians can only prescribe a thirty-day supply of the drug, so you need to return to the office monthly to get a new prescription.

Antibiotics for Acne and Rosacea

Antibiotics work for pimples and painful lumps that develop from acne and rosacea, but they don't remove blackheads and whiteheads. They are typically prescribed if the condition fails to respond to topical treatments, if the patient develops painful lumps under the skin, or if scarring arises. Doxycycline (Adoxa, Doryx, Oracea, and Periostat), tetracycline, and minocycline (Minocin and Solodyne) are the most commonly prescribed antibiotics. They work by killing bacteria that live in the hair follicles and cause acne and rosacea. They also have special anti-inflammatory properties. For the antibiotics to work most effectively, patients must take them every day, and results are typically not seen for a few weeks. Antibiotics work better and better over a two-month time frame, at which point they will be working their best. At the two-month time point, you can expect about 30 percent improvement. Therefore, if you started with one hundred bumps on the skin, you can expect to see approximately seventy bumps at the two-month time point; the exact number may vary between days. If you stop using the antibiotic, you may gradually lose the improvement you achieved, but if you continue the treatment you should maintain your progress.

Doxycycline may be taken once or twice a day with food to avoid an upset stomach. Tetracycline may be taken once or twice a day, and it should be taken one hour before or two hours after meals, because food will block the body's ability to absorb the drug. Minocycline may be taken once or twice a day with food to avoid an upset stomach. Do not take any of these antibiotics within one to two hours of consuming dairy products, antacids (Tums), or supplements containing calcium, magnesium, iron, or zinc, because they will block the absorption of the drug into your system.

Overall, antibiotics are safe, but as with any drug, side effects may occur. If you think you are experiencing side effects, stop the drug and call your doctor. Antibiotics can make your skin sensitive to the sun, so you may need to wear a hat or apply sunscreen over your acne creams before going outside. Use sunscreens that are oil free, or noncomedogenic, which means they won't cause acne. Other possible side effects include headaches, dizziness, stomach upset, and diarrhea. They could also cause heartburn, particularly if you take the pill and immediately lie down. Therefore, take your nighttime dose at least one hour before bedtime to give it a chance to absorb into your stomach. Antibiotics can also cause yeast infections, so call your doctor if you experience itching or discharge. Finally, antibiotics can cause birth defects and could theoretically make birth control pills less effective, so use two forms of contraception if you are sexually active. Women should also stop the medicine if they become pregnant.

Pharmaceutical companies have developed new, alternative forms of antibiotics to help reduce side effects and add convenience. However, they may be expensive. Adoxa is a form of doxycycline that only needs to be taken once daily. Doryx is a coated form of doxycycline that is gentler on the stomach and is taken once daily. Oracea is a form of low dose doxycycline that does not kill bacteria and is taken once daily. Periostat is another form of low-dose doxycycline that does not kill bacteria and is taken twice daily. Finally, Solodyn is a slow-release form of minocycline that is taken once a day and has fewer side effects than standard minocycline.

CellCept (Mycophenolate Mofetil)

CellCept is a pill taken for skin conditions caused by an overactive immune system. It takes a month or more to kick in and works by suppressing the immune system. CellCept is often prescribed with prednisone, which acts must faster and must be used initially to get the condition under control quickly. The prednisone dose can then be lowered over the long term. I start patients on a low dose of CellCept and increase the dose gradually. Once they are on a good dose of CellCept and the skin condition is in remission, I try to reduce the dose of prednisone. Then once the dose of prednisone is negligible, the dose of CellCept may be reduced for as long as the skin condition remains in remission.

Periodic blood tests are needed to help avoid side effects during therapy. For example, CellCept could cause a drop in red blood cell counts, white blood cell counts, and platelets. Therefore, you need a complete blood cell count before starting treatment, and once you're on the drug, this test must be repeated every two weeks for the first two months, then monthly thereafter.

CellCept could also cause liver inflammation. Therefore, you need a blood test for markers of liver inflammation before starting treatment, and this test must be repeated one month after starting the medicine, then every three months thereafter.

CellCept works by suppressing the immune system, thereby increasing your risk for infections. You therefore need a purified protein derivative skin test before starting treatment to make sure tuberculosis is not hiding anywhere in your body. If you develop an infection on CellCept, call your doctor because you may need to stop the medicine and take antibiotics.

The immunosuppressive nature of CellCept also makes it unsafe to receive live vaccines during therapy. Before you start treatment, your doctor should administer any live vaccines you may need in the foreseeable future.

CellCept could also increase your risk for cancer, but this is unlikely with the lower doses of CellCept usually prescribed by dermatologists. Other specialists, such as transplant surgeons, prescribe CellCept at much higher doses. Your risk for developing skin cancer could also rise while on CellCept, so visit your dermatologist for any suspicious new or changing skin growths. Avoiding excessive sun exposure may also reduce your risk for developing skin cancer. For advice on sun protection, see the beginning of the essay "Skin Aging: Prevention and Treatment" in Part I of this book.

Finally, do not get pregnant while taking CellCept or start the drug if you plan to get pregnant soon since it could cause birth defects.

Corticosteroid Creams

Corticosteroid creams are used for a variety of skin conditions caused by an overactive immune system, such as psoriasis, eczema, and allergic contact dermatitis. These creams work by suppressing the immune system where directly applied. They are not considered cures, however, because when they are stopped, the underlying condition may return.

Commonly prescribed corticosteroid creams include hydrocortisone, triamcinalone, and clobetasol, in order from weakest to strongest. Clobetasol cream works the fastest and hydrocortisone the slowest, with triamcinalone in between.

When used appropriately, these creams do not usually cause side effects. Skin atrophy, which means thin skin, is the most common adverse effect reported. If you use a corticosteroid cream for several months, your skin may start to thin out and appear shiny and wrinkled. Tiny blood vessels may appear on the skin's surface. In many cases, atrophy resolves when treatment is discontinued.

To avoid skin atrophy, apply the cream to the rash only, not to normal-looking skin around the rash. Moreover, stop the cream when itching and redness largely resolve. A moisturizer is often appropriate to use during this break. If the rash recurs, though, it is often acceptable to restart the corticosteroid cream.

If the redness or itching fails to respond to treatment after a few weeks, it may not work at all, and you should consider returning to the dermatologist for reevaluation. If the redness or itching does respond but you need to use the cream daily for months with no breaks in order to maintain relief, you may need an alternative treatment to avoid skin atrophy or other side effects. Elidel (pimecrolimus cream) and Protopic (tacrolimus ointment) are nonsteroidal anti-inflammatory creams you could try that will not cause skin atrophy after prolonged use. Elidel and Protopic are typically far more expensive to buy than hydrocortisone, triamcinalone, and clobetasol creams, which are available in generic formulations. Narrowband ultraviolet light type B phototherapy may also be appropriate in these difficult cases. See Part II of this book for more information about this treatment option.

Cyclosporine

Cyclosporine is a pill used for skin conditions caused by an overactive immune system, such as psoriasis, eczema, and hives. It works by suppressing the immune system.

Periodic tests are needed to help avoid side effects during therapy. For example, cyclosporine can affect the kidneys, so you need a urine and blood test for kidney function before starting treatment, and these tests must be repeated every two weeks for the first few months, then monthly after that.

Cyclosporine can also alter your uric acid and electrolyte levels. Therefore, you need a baseline uric acid and electrolyte panel before starting the medicine. This test is repeated every two weeks for the first few months on the drug, then monthly.

Patients could develop elevated cholesterol during therapy, so you also need a fasting cholesterol test before starting treatment. After you start on the medicine, this test is repeated every two weeks for the first few months, then monthly thereafter.

In addition, blood pressure could rise during treatment, so you need a blood pressure check before starting the medicine. Once you are on the drug, this test is repeated every two weeks for the first few months, then monthly after that.

Cyclosporine works by suppressing your immune system, thereby increasing your risk for infections. Therefore, you need a purified protein derivative skin test before initiating treatment to make sure tuberculosis is not hiding anywhere in your body. If you develop an infection during treatment, call your doctor, because you may need to stop the drug and take antibiotics. The immunosuppressive nature of cyclosporine also makes it unsafe to receive live vaccines during therapy. Your doctor should administer any live vaccines you may need in the foreseeable future before you start treatment.

Cyclosporine could increase your risk for cancer, but this is unlikely on the low doses of cyclosporine usually prescribed by dermatologists. Other specialists, such as transplant surgeons, prescribe cyclosporine at much higher doses to treat other conditions. Your risk for skin cancer may also rise on cyclosporine, so visit your dermatologist for any suspicious new or changing skin growths. Avoiding excessive sun exposure may also reduce your risk for developing skin cancer. For advice on sun protection, see the beginning of the essay "Skin Aging: Prevention and Treatment" in Part I of this book.

Cyclosporine can interact with many other medicines, so tell your dermatologist about every medicine you take, and tell your other doctors you are on cyclosporine before they start you on any new medicines.

To learn more about cyclosporine, psoriasis patients should join the National Psoriasis Foundation, visit its website at www.psoriasis.org, and follow the links for treatments.

Dapsone

Dapsone is a pill taken for certain skin conditions such as leukocytoclastic vasculitis and pyoderma gangrenosum, which are caused by immune cells called neutrophils. Dapsone works by suppressing the neutrophils.

Periodic blood tests are needed to prevent side effects during treatment. For example, dapsone could lower blood cell counts in patients with a deficiency in an enzyme called glucose-6-phosphate dehydrogenase. Your enzyme levels will, therefore, be measured before initiating therapy.

Dapsone could also lower blood cell counts in patients without an enzyme deficiency, so you need a complete blood cell count before starting treatment. Once you are on the drug, this test is repeated weekly for four weeks, then every two weeks for eight weeks, then every three months thereafter. If your red cell counts drop, you could feel tired, and if your white cell counts fall, you could get an infection.

Patients could also develop liver inflammation, so you need a blood test for markers of liver inflammation before starting treatment. This test is repeated every three months once on the drug.

Finally, you need a urinalysis or kidney function test before starting treatment and, once on the drug, every three months thereafter.

If you develop a fever and a rash on dapsone, please call your doctor immediately, because serious drug reactions have been reported. There is also a small chance that dapsone can affect your nerves, so tell your doctor if you develop hand or leg weakness.

Enbrel, Humira, and Remicade

Enbrel (etanercept) treats psoriasis and psoriatic arthritis. It works by suppressing the immune system. Enbrel is administered at home by subcutaneous injections, either once a week or twice a week. It is typically prescribed for psoriasis not easily controlled with creams or if narrowband ultraviolet light type B phototherapy is not an option. It is also used for psoriatic arthritis uncontrolled by nonsteroidal anti-inflammatory medicines. Enbrel does much more than these medicines for psoriatic arthritis. Anti-inflammatory medicines only cover up pain and stiffness, but Enbrel may halt the destructive progression of the arthritis, which could otherwise lead to disability. It takes a few weeks to kick in, but is not fully functional for six months. Many patients stay on Enbrel for years if they tolerate it.

Enbrel is very effective for psoriasis and psoriatic arthritis, but like any drug, it can have side effects. The most common are injection-site reactions—some redness and tenderness at the site of administration. Ice, Tylenol (acetaminophen), and Benadryl (diphenhydramine) are helpful treatments for these reactions.

Enbrel works by suppressing the immune system, thereby increasing your risk for infections. You therefore need a purified protein derivative skin test before starting treatment to make sure tuberculosis is not hiding anywhere inside your body. Moreover, if you expect to be in contact with tuberculosis patients while on therapy, this drug is not for you. Finally, if you develop an infection on Enbrel, call your doctor, because you may need to stop the drug and take antibiotics.

The immunosuppressive nature of Enbrel also makes it unsafe to receive live vaccines during therapy. Before you start treatment, your doctor should administer any live vaccines you may need in the foreseeable future.

Other rare side effects include a syndrome that acts like lupus, a syndrome that acts similar to multiple sclerosis, and congestive heart failure. Finally, there is a theoretical risk of developing lymphoma or other cancer. Doctors do not really know if this risk is real or not—some studies show there is a risk, and other studies show that there is no risk. Psoriasis by itself could increase your risk for developing a lymphoma.

Many patients use Enbrel for years and years with no problem, but if you stop using Enbrel, your psoriasis or arthritis may come back. Indeed, there is no true cure for psoriasis. Therefore, if you decide at some point to stop using Enbrel, it may be wise to start a substitute treatment. Typically, during this period of changing remedies, it's a good idea to have topical corticosteroid creams and nonsteroidal anti-inflammatory drugs around to treat any symptoms that come back.

Humira (adalimumab) works like Enbrel, but it is injected at home every other week. It is somewhat more effective than Enbrel, but chances for side effects are somewhat higher, too. Remicade (infliximab) works like Enbrel and Humira, but it must be infused through an intravenous line in a physician's office every few weeks at first, then every few months. It is more effective than Enbrel and Humira, but chances for side effects are somewhat higher. To learn more about Enbrel, Humira, and Remicade, join the National Psoriasis Foundation, visit its website at www.psoriasis.org, and follow the links for treatments.

Imuran (Azathioprine)

Imuran is a pill used for skin conditions caused by an overactive immune system, such as pemphigus, bullous pemphigoid, eczema, or vasculitis. It takes a month or longer to begin working and functions by suppressing the immune system. Imuran is often prescribed with prednisone, which acts must faster and must be used to initially get the condition under control quickly. The prednisone dose can then be lowered over the long term. I start patients on a low dose of Imuran and increase the dose gradually. Once the patient is on a good dose of Imuran and the skin condition is in remission, I try to reduce the dose of prednisone. Then, once the dose of prednisone is negligible, the dose of Imuran may be reduced for as long as the skin condition remains in remission.

Periodic blood tests are needed to avoid side effects during treatment. For example, Imuran can lower blood cell counts in patients with a deficiency in an enzyme called thiopurine methyltransferase. Your enzyme levels will therefore be measured before initiating therapy.

Even patients without an enzyme deficiency could develop low levels of red blood cells, white blood cells, or platelets during therapy. You therefore need a complete blood cell count before starting treatment, and once you are on the drug, this test is repeated every other week for the first two months, then every two months thereafter. If your red cell count declines, you may feel tired; if your white cell count drops, you could get an infection; and if your platelet levels fall, you could develop nosebleeds or reddish spots on your skin.

In rare cases patients develop liver inflammation during therapy, so you need a blood test for markers of liver inflammation before starting the drug. After the medicine is started, this test is repeated every other week for the first two months, then every two months thereafter.

Imuran works by suppressing the immune system and thereby increases your risk for infections. Therefore, you need a purified protein derivative skin test before starting treatment to make sure tuberculosis is not hiding anywhere in your body. If you develop an infection on Imuran, call your doctor because you may need to stop the drug and take antibiotics.

The immunosuppressive nature of Imuran may also increase your risk for developing cancer, but this is unlikely with the lower doses usually prescribed by dermatologists. Other specialists, such as transplant surgeons, prescribe Imuran at much higher doses. Imuran could also increase your risk for skin cancer, so visit your dermatologist for any suspicious new or changing skin growths. Avoiding excessive sun exposure may also reduce your risk for developing skin cancer. For advice on sun protection, see the beginning of the essay "Skin Aging: Prevention and Treatment" in Part I of this book.

Do not get pregnant while taking Imuran or start the drug if you plan to get pregnant soon, since it could cause birth defects. Finally, Imuran can cause a serious type of skin rash that often presents with fever. If this happens, call your dermatologist immediately, because you may need treatment and may need to stop the drug.

Methotrexate

Methotrexate is used for skin conditions caused by an overactive immune system, like psoriasis and bullous pemphigoid. It works by suppressing the immune system and is taken in a pill form once a week. Results are typically seen a few weeks after starting the medicine.

Periodic blood tests are needed to avoid side effects during treatment. For example, methotrexate can cause liver inflammation, so you need a blood test for markers of liver inflammation before starting treatment. This test is repeated weekly during the first few months of treatment. To avoid liver toxicity, do not drink alcohol while on the medicine. If you crave alcohol, this medicine is not for you. Finally, if you stay on methotrexate for a few years, you may need a liver biopsy to confirm that the drug is not affecting your liver. Of course, you may stop the medicine and find a substitute before needing a liver biopsy.

Methotrexate can also lower levels of your red blood cells, white blood cells, and platelets. Therefore, you need a complete blood cell count before starting the drug. This test is repeated weekly during the first few months of treatment. Taking medicines that interact with methotrexate could substantially add to the risk for this side effect. Therefore, avoid medicines that interact with methotrexate—especially over-the-counter pain medicines—like aspirin, ibuprofen, and naprosyn.

If your red cell count drops, you may feel tired, and if your platelet levels fall, you may notice tiny pink spots on your skin or develop nosebleeds. In addition, you could develop an infection if your white cell count declines. To help prevent methotrexate from lowering blood cell counts, you may need a folate supplement every day, except the one day of the week that you take methotrexate.

Methotrexate works by suppressing the immune system, thereby increasing your risk for infections. Therefore, you need a purified protein derivative skin test before starting treatment to make sure tuberculosis is not hiding anywhere in your body. If you develop an infection during treatment, call your doctor because you may need to stop the medicine and take antibiotics.

The immunosuppressive nature of methotrexate may also increase your risk for cancer, but this is unlikely on the low doses usually prescribed for dermatologic use. Other specialists prescribe methotrexate at much higher doses.

Finally, do not get pregnant while taking methotrexate or start the drug if you plan to get pregnant soon, since it could cause birth defects.

Some Drugs that Interact With Methotrexate

Serious side effects, even death, may result from taking other drugs that interact with methotrexate. If you start taking this medicine, inform your other doctors so they don't accidentally prescribe you a medicine that interacts with it. Nonprescription drugs could also interact with methotrexate, so you must take responsibility and make sure no drug you take will interact with it. Please ask your doctor or pharmacist if you have any questions. Listed below are some common drugs that interact with methotrexate. This list is not complete—there are other pharmaceuticals that may not be safe to take with it.

Nonsteroidal Anti-inflammatory Drugs

Ibuprofen (Advil, Motrin)
Indomethacin (Indocin)
Naprosyn (Aleve, Naproxen)
Salicylates (aspirin)

Antibiotics

Ciprofloxacin
Penicillins
Tetracyclines
Trimethoprim-sulfamethoxazole (Bactrim)

Other Drugs

Barbituates
Colchicine (Colcrys)
Dipyridamole (Persantine)
Ethanol (alcohol)
Furosemide (Lasix)
Hydrochlorothiazide
Phenytoin (Dilantin)
Probenecid
Sulfonylureas

Narrowband Ultraviolet Light Type B Phototherapy

Narrowband ultraviolet light type B phototherapy is typically used for skin conditions caused by an overactive immune system, such as psoriasis, vitiligo, and eczema, but it can be used for other conditions, too, such as mycosis fungoides and itching. Treatments may work by suppressing immune cells in the skin. Phototherapy units emit light in a narrow band of wavelengths, approximately 311 to 313 nanometers. These devices are not tanning booths, however. They are medical instruments designed to emit safe forms of light.

Treatments are often administered at a clinic two or three times a week, but never on back-to-back days. You start on a low dose of light, and every time you return, the dose may be increased, depending on how you tolerate and respond to therapy. It usually takes only a few minutes to receive your dose of light. Patients who cannot attend frequent clinic sessions may be prescribed a phototherapy device for home use.

Treatments for psoriasis may work better if immediately prior to sessions you coat your rash with mineral oil, which can be purchased at the pharmacy. During light treatments, your face and private areas are protected. In most cases, light therapy continues until your skin condition resolves. Then, the frequency of treatments is tapered down or stopped altogether, depending on your skin condition.

The most common side effects include itching and burning, which may necessitate reducing the dose of light you receive. Signs of skin aging, such as wrinkling, are also a potential effect of long-term use. To date there is no definitive proof that narrow band ultraviolet light type B phototherapy causes skin cancer.

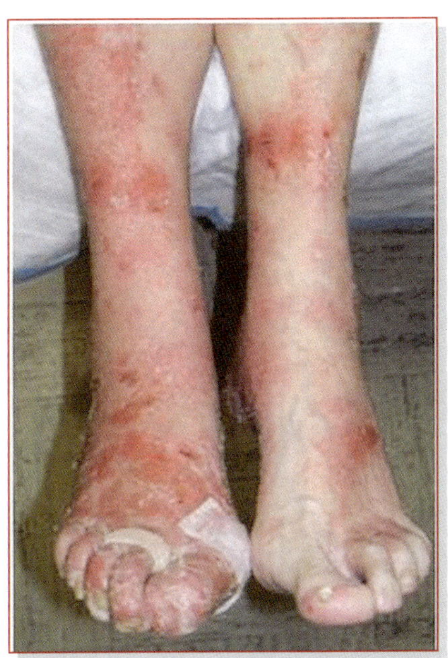

Severe psoriasis

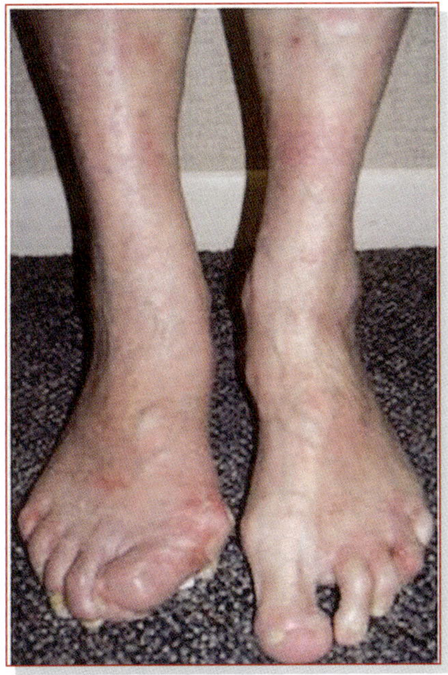

Improvement after treatment with narrowband ultraviolet light type B phototherapy and Humira

Plaquenil (Hydroxychloroquine)

Plaquenil is a medicine most commonly used for skin conditions caused by an overactive immune system, such as lupus and lichen planus.

Periodic blood tests are needed to help avoid side effects during treatment. For example, plaquenil could lower blood cell counts in patients with a deficiency in an enzyme called glucose-6-phosphate dehydrogenase. Your enzyme levels may therefore be measured before initiating therapy.

Plaquenil could also cause lower blood cell counts in patients without an enzyme deficiency, so you need a complete blood cell count before starting treatment. This test is repeated monthly for the first three months on the drug, then every four to six months thereafter.

Patients could also develop liver inflammation on the drug, so you need a blood test for markers of liver inflammation before starting treatment. Once you are on the drug, this test is repeated in one month, three months, and then every four to six months thereafter.

Plaquenil can also affect your vision, so you need a baseline eye exam to make sure plaquenil will be safe to start. A slit lamp, fundascopic, and visual field test should be performed. These tests are typically repeated every twelve months while on the drug. Alert your doctor if you develop blurred vision, have discomfort upon looking into bright light, or see halos around lights.

Finally, some patients on the drug may develop a bluish color on their shins, face, or nails, so alert your doctor if this happens. This is a cosmetic issue, but may be disconcerting.

Prednisone

Prednisone is a pill taken for skin conditions caused by an overactive immune system. It works by suppressing the immune system. When patients without medical problems take low to moderate doses for short periods of time—three weeks or less—prednisone often causes no problems. More caution is needed for patients with certain medical problems or if prednisone will be continued for months.

Patients with specific medical problems and patients who require more than three weeks of therapy need periodic tests to help avoid side effects. For example, prednisone could cause alterations in electrolyte levels, cholesterol levels, and blood glucose levels. Therefore, you may need a fasting blood test before starting treatment, and once you are on the drug this test must be repeated in one month, then every three months thereafter.

Patients requiring more than three weeks of prednisone could also develop bone degeneration. Therefore, you may require a test for osteoporosis, called a DEXA scan, before starting treatment, and this test is repeated every six to twelve months thereafter. You may also need to take vitamin D, calcium, and possibly Fosamax (alendronate) to prevent osteoporosis.

Blood pressure could also rise on prednisone, so you may need a blood pressure measurement before starting treatment. This test is repeated every other month while on the medicine.

Prednisone could also cause or worsen cataracts and glaucoma, so an eye exam may be needed before starting treatment. This test is repeated every six to twelve months thereafter.

Prednisone works by suppressing the immune system, thereby increasing your risk for infections. Patients requiring more than three weeks of treatment therefore need a purified protein derivative skin test to make sure tuberculosis is not hiding anywhere in their bodies. Once on prednisone, if you develop any kind of infection, call your doctor because you may need antibiotics.

Other possible side effects include stomach upset or even ulcers if prednisone is taken with nonsteroidal anti-inflammatory medicines (aspirin, ibuprofen, or naprosyn), emotional agitation, suppression of the adrenal gland in long-term users, and a condition called Cushing's disease in long-term users.

If you will be on prednisone for multiple months, you may require a steroid-sparing medicine to reduce your reliance on prednisone. Common steroid-sparing pharmaceuticals include Imuran (azathioprine), CellCept (mycophenolate mofetil), and methotrexate. The ultimate goal is often to taper down and, hopefully, discontinue prednisone, while keeping you on steroid-sparing medicines for the long haul.

Soriatane (Acitretin)

Soriatane is most commonly prescribed for psoriasis, although it may be helpful for other conditions, such as lichen planus. It comes in pill form and is taken daily. Unlike some other treatments for psoriasis, Soriatane does not suppress the immune system and therefore does not increase one's risk for infections or malignancy.

Soriatane can cause birth defects, so women of childbearing potential need pregnancy tests before, during, and after treatment. In addition, these women should not drink alcohol during treatment, because a single drink could cause a chemical reaction that makes Soriatane persist in the body for years, making it unsafe to bear children for three years after stopping the medicine.

Periodic blood tests are needed to help avoid side effects. For example, Soriatane could raise your cholesterol values, in rare cases high enough to inflame your pancreas. Therefore you need a fasting blood test before starting the medicine, and once on the drug this test is repeated monthly for three months, and then once every three months.

Soriatane could also cause liver inflammation, so you need a blood test for markers of liver inflammation before starting the medicine. After initiating therapy, this test is repeated monthly for three months, and then every three months.

A complete blood cell count and a blood test for kidney function are also needed before starting the medicine. Once you are on the drug these tests are repeated monthly for three months, then every three months.

Finally, some patients who take Soriatane for very long periods may develop tender bone abnormalities called osteophytes. For this reason, baseline X-rays are sometimes considered before starting the medicine. Tell your doctor if you develop aches and pains while on Soriatane.

Stelara (Ustekinumab)

Stelara treats psoriasis and psoriatic arthritis by suppressing the immune system. It is very effective and works rather quickly—you should notice results within a few weeks. Stelara is administered in the office by a member of the dermatology staff with an injection, which is repeated in a month, then once every three months thereafter.

Stelara works by suppressing the immune system and thereby increases your risk for infections. Therefore, you need a purified protein derivative skin test before starting treatment to make sure tuberculosis is not hiding anywhere in your body. If you develop an infection while on the medicine, call your doctor because you may need antibiotics.

Finally, the immunosuppressive nature of Stelara makes it unsafe to receive live vaccines during treatment. Your doctor should therefore administer any live vaccines you may need in the foreseeable future before you start the medicine.

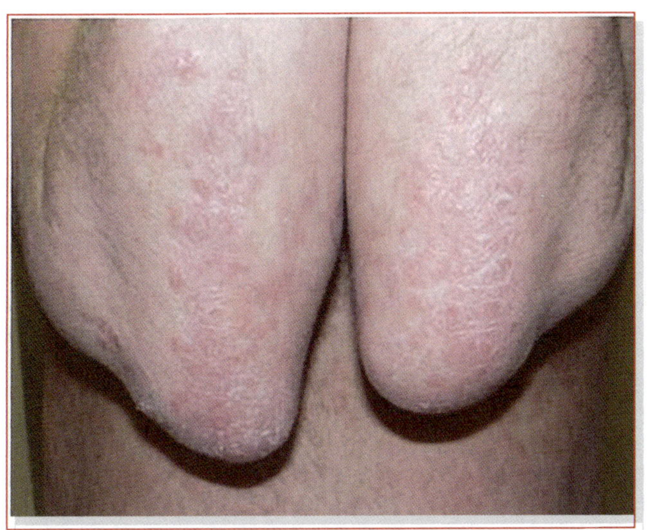

Psoriasis of the elbows

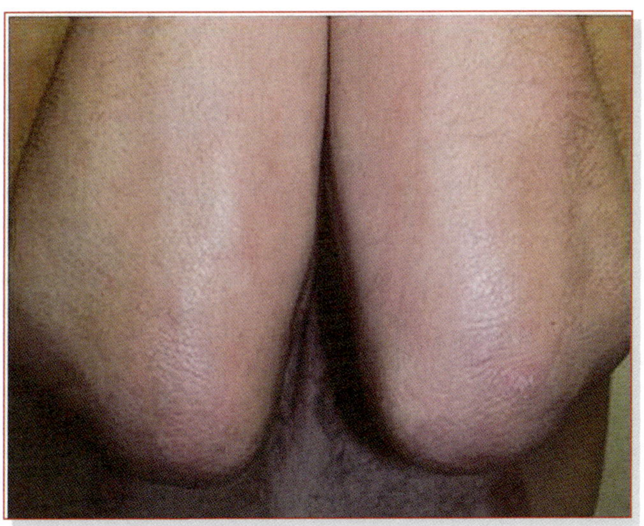

Improvement from Stelara and Soriatane

Part I I I
Cosmetic Treatments

Blepharoplasty

Blepharoplasty is a cosmetic surgery technique that removes excess skin from the upper eyelids that can cause a person to appear tired and older. Therefore, after the procedure, patients typically look younger and more awake.

Blepharoplasty is performed in the office and requires only local anesthesia. Hence, you are awake the entire time, and the procedure requires only a few hours. Arrange to have someone drive you home on the day of the procedure, and prepare to return in one week for suture removal. Finally, expect about a week of some swelling and bruising, so consider taking one week off from work if you would be concerned about your appearance.

To decrease discomfort and anxiety, consider taking Valium (5 mg) forty-five minutes before the procedure. Tell your doctor if you wish to take an anti-anxiety medicine. If you do take Valium, you will need a ride to and from the office.

Do not discontinue blood thinners if they have been prescribed by your physician, especially if you have had a heart attack, stroke, or clot. Aspirin, Coumadin (warfarin), Plavix (clopidogrel), and Pradaxa (dabigatran) are common blood thinners. If you have never had a heart attack, stroke, or blood clot, and you are taking aspirin for other reasons, you may consider stopping it two weeks before surgery and restarting it one week after surgery. Ask your doctor if this is acceptable in your situation before making a decision.

Nonsteroidal anti-inflammatory medicines commonly used for headaches and joint pain may increase your risk for bleeding. These medicines include diclofenac (Arthrotec), ibuprofen (Advil and Motrin), indomethacin (Indocin), meloxicam (Mobic), naprosyn (Aleve or Naproxen), and sulindac (Clinoril). If you have a healthy liver and kidneys, Tylenol is a preferred pain medicine that will not increase your risk for bleeding.

Other supplements that may increase your risk for bleeding include vitamin E, ginkgo biloba, garlic, glucosamine, and fish oil. Please avoid these supplements for up to two weeks before and one week after the procedure.

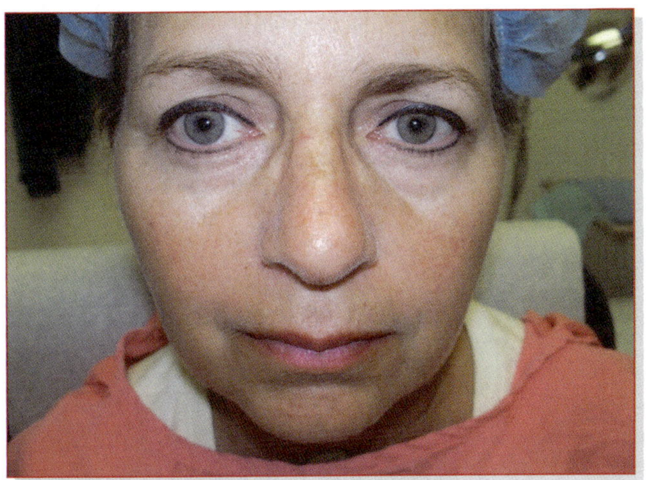

Hooding of the upper eyelids

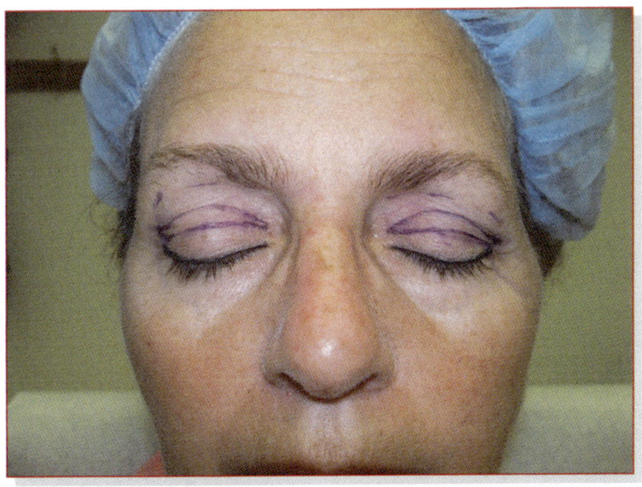

Skin to be removed during blepharoplasty outlined with a felt-tipped pen

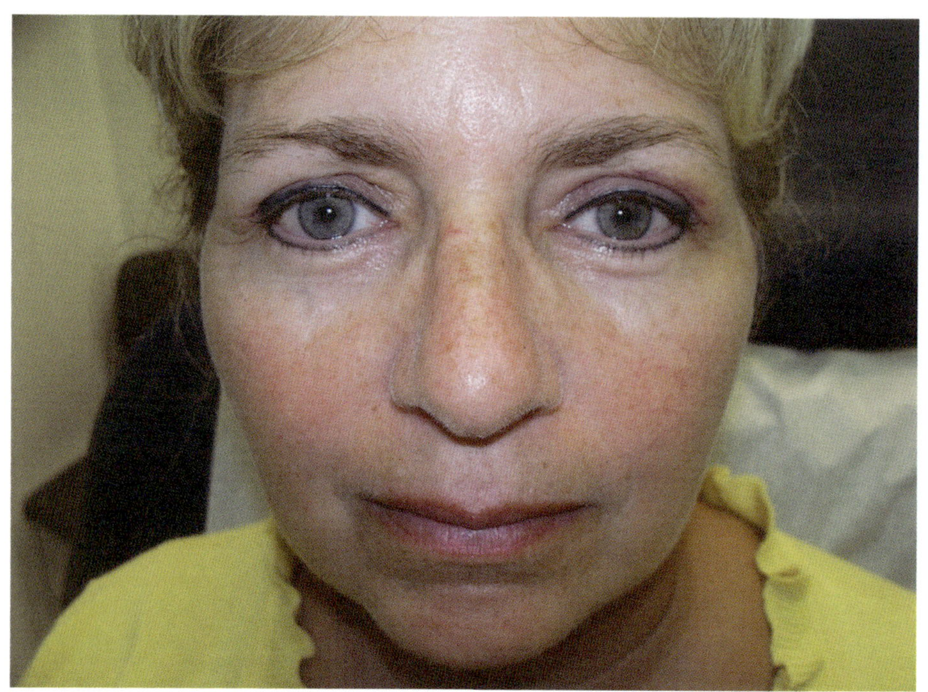

Patient one week after blepharoplasty with hooding corrected

Skin Care Instructions for After a Blepharoplasty

Apply an ice pack or cold pack for the first forty-eight hours to reduce swelling and bruising. A mild amount of discomfort is normal when the lidocaine wears off. If you have a normally functioning liver, consider taking two extra-strength Tylenol every four to six hours. It's a good idea to take some as soon as you get home from the procedure, even before the lidocaine wears off completely.

Apply erythromycin ointment to the surgical site on your eyelids three times a day: morning, noon, and nighttime. Showering is permissible, but do not scrub your eyelids in the shower. Also, do not perform any exercise or activity that could raise your blood pressure. A rise in your blood pressure could increase your chance of bleeding. Finally, call your doctor if there is any excessive bleeding, swelling, discomfort, or change in your vision.

Botox (Botulinum Toxin)

Botox is FDA-approved for the treatment of facial wrinkles that form above the nose due to muscle contractions when a person frowns. It is a clear fluid that is injected into the affected muscles and paralyzes them, making the wrinkles go away. Treatments are well tolerated and typically safe when used for cosmetic purposes. Results may be seen within a few days and last approximately three months.

PRETREATMENT DIRECTIONS

Botox works very well for wrinkles caused by muscle contraction, called dynamic wrinkles. Treatments do not, however, remove lines caused by gravity or sun damage, called static wrinkles. Therefore, some types of wrinkles will not respond to Botox. These persistent lines can be treated with other methods, such as fillers (Radiesse, Juvederm, and Restylane), laser resurfacing, chemical peels, and tretinoin cream. See Part III of this book to learn more about some of these treatments.

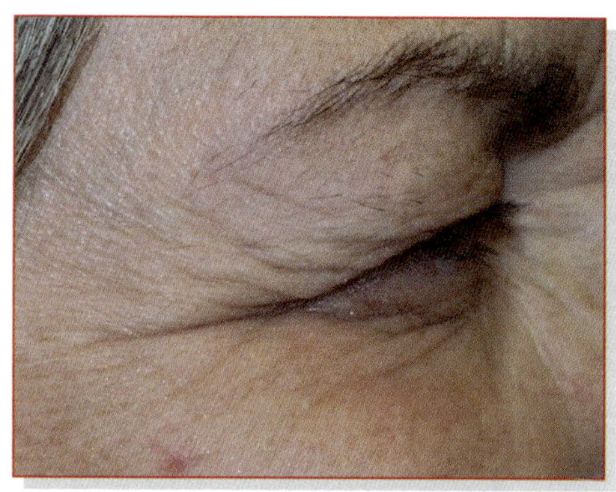

Squinting before Botox treatments

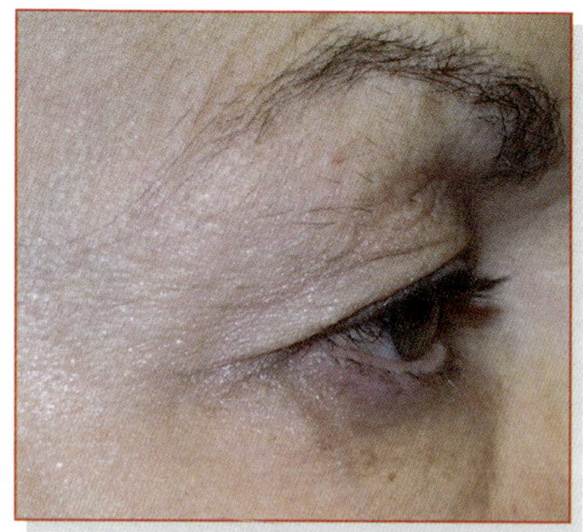

Squinting inhibited
after Botox treatments

Part III Cosmetic Treatments

Chemical Peel—Medium Depth

Medium-depth chemical peels are used for a variety of skin conditions, including actinic keratoses, fine wrinkles, acne scarring, small growths, and lentigines (liver spots and sun spots). Medium-depth peels treat the epidermis and some of the superficial dermis. Jessner's solution followed by 35 percent trichloroacetic acid is used for these peels, which have an excellent safety record.

PRETREATMENT DIRECTIONS

1. During the treatment, your skin develops a white frost, which resolves within hours. Your skin in the treated area will also begin to peel off within days and continue peeling for approximately one to two weeks. Therefore, if you have an important social engagement within the next few days, defer treatment until a later date.

2. Use sunscreen with a sun protection factor that prevents tanning and burning. Too much sun before a peel can lead to brown splotches after the peel.

3. If you have ever had fever blisters or cold sores, consider taking Valtrex (valacyclovir 500 mg twice daily), beginning the day before the peel and continuing for two weeks after the peel. Cold sores and fever blisters are caused by a herpes virus, and skin trauma from the peel could cause the condition to recur.

4. Do not apply moisturizers to your face the morning of the peel because they reduce the peel's effectiveness.

5. To decrease discomfort and swelling, consider taking aspirin (325 mg) one hour before the peel and then every four hours

for the rest of the day. Ask your doctor if this optional step is appropriate for you.

6. To decrease discomfort and anxiety, consider taking Valium (5 mg) forty-five minutes before the peel. Tell your doctor if you wish to take an anti-anxiety medicine. If you do take Valium, you will need a ride to and from the office. This step is optional.

POSTTREATMENT DIRECTIONS

1. Apply a moisturizer, such as Aquaphor, until all peeling is complete, approximately seven days after treatment. If scabs and crusts form, apply a moisturizer until they resolve. Do not pick the scabs and crusts off.

2. Consider using Cetaphil liquid cleanser as your soap. Patients can resume wearing makeup in seven to fourteen days, when the skin has stopped peeling.

3. Limit your sun exposure to help prevent the recurrence of actinic keratoses, fine wrinkles, and brown spots that were treated by the peel. For advice on sun protection, see the beginning of the essay "Skin Aging: Prevention and Treatment" in Part I of this book.

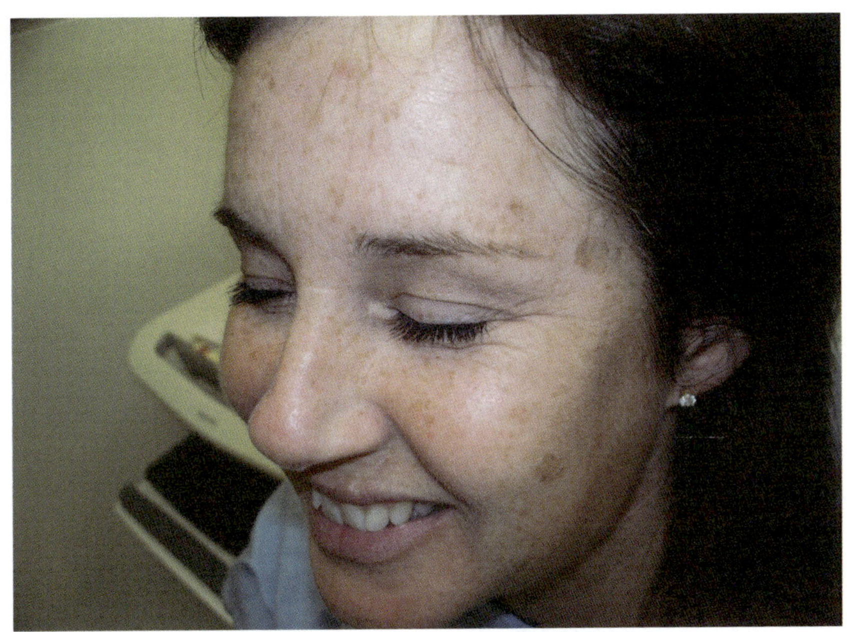

Multiple lentigines on the face

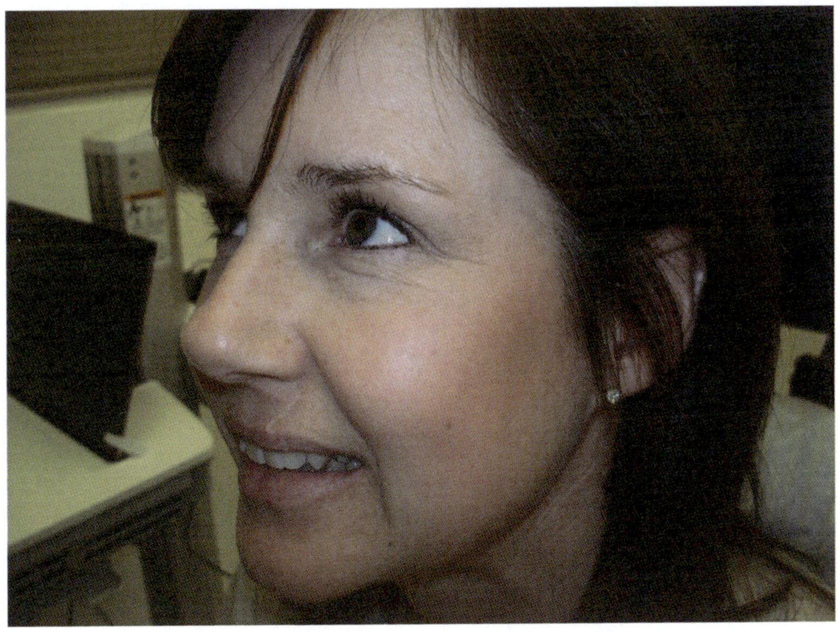

Cosmetic result after medium-depth chemical peel

Chemical Peel—Superficial

Superficial chemical peels are used for a variety of skin conditions, including very fine wrinkles, acne, lentigines (sun spots and liver spots), and melasma. Superficial peels treat the epidermis. Many types of chemicals are used for peeling, including glycolic acid, Jessner's solution, and trichloroacetic acid. They have an excellent safety record and require no anesthesia. All skin colors may be treated with rapid healing and minimal downtime. Some clinical benefit is attained with a single peel, but getting repeated peels every three to six weeks provides more cumulative benefits.

PRETREATMENT DIRECTIONS

1. Your skin may not actually peel following treatment, but it may appear pink for a few hours to days. Therefore, if you have an important social engagement within the next few days, defer treatment until a later date.

2. Use sunscreen with a sun protection factor that prevents tanning and burning. Too much sun before a peel can lead to brown splotches after the peel.

3. If you have ever had fever blisters or cold sores, consider taking Valtrex (valacyclovir, 500 mg twice daily) beginning the day before the peel and continuing for two weeks after the peel. Cold sores and fever blisters are caused by a herpes virus, and skin trauma from the peel could cause the condition to recur.

4. Do not apply moisturizers to your face the morning of the procedure because they reduce the peel's effectiveness.

POSTTREATMENT DIRECTIONS

1. Apply a moisturizer, such as Aquaphor, until all peeling is complete.

2. Consider using Cetaphil liquid cleanser as your soap until the skin is completely rejuvenated, then resume your regular skin care routine.

3. Limit your sun exposure to help prevent the recurrence of fine wrinkles and brown spots that were treated by the peel. For advice on sun protection, see the beginning of the essay "Skin Aging: Prevention and Treatment" in Part I of this book.

Earlobe Repair

Years of wearing earrings can stretch your earlobes to the point of tearing. It may be preferable to repair the holes before they tear. The dermatologist first injects lidocaine around the holes to numb the area. He or she then removes the skin lining the rim around the hole. This procedure is needed to create fresh skin edges that the doctor can then permanently bring together with sutures. Once the sutures are removed, you may consider piercing the earlobe again in a different location.

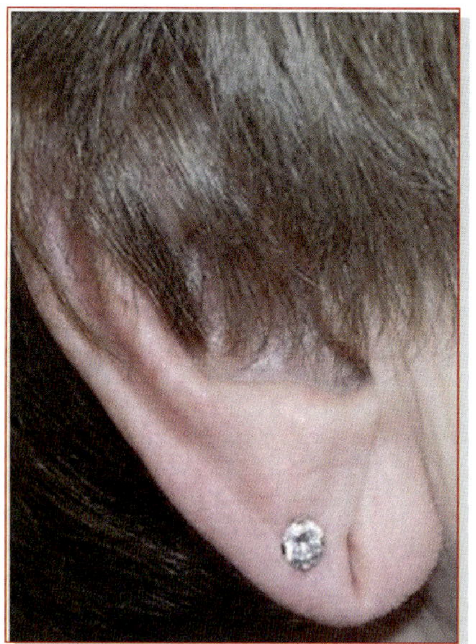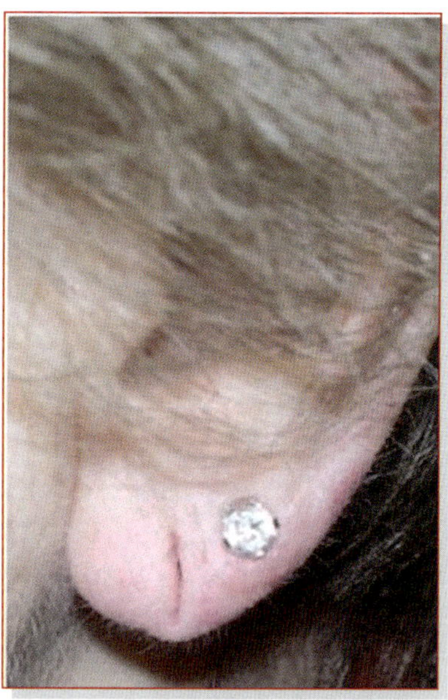

Elongated, stretched earlobe holes in need of repair

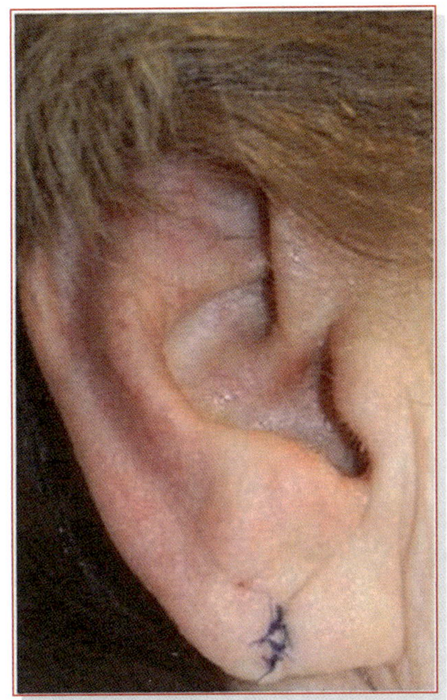
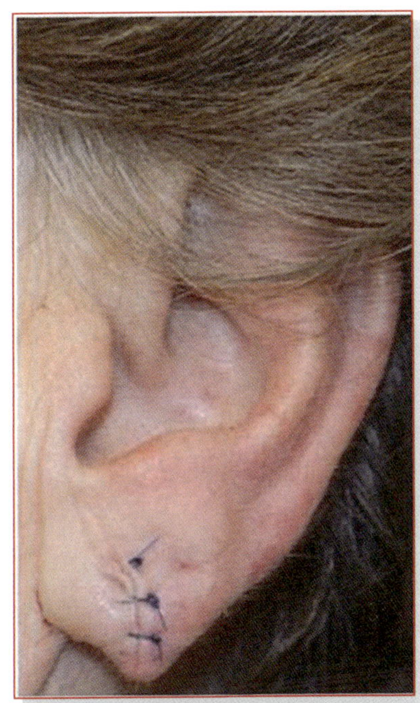

Earlobe holes surgically repaired and sutured

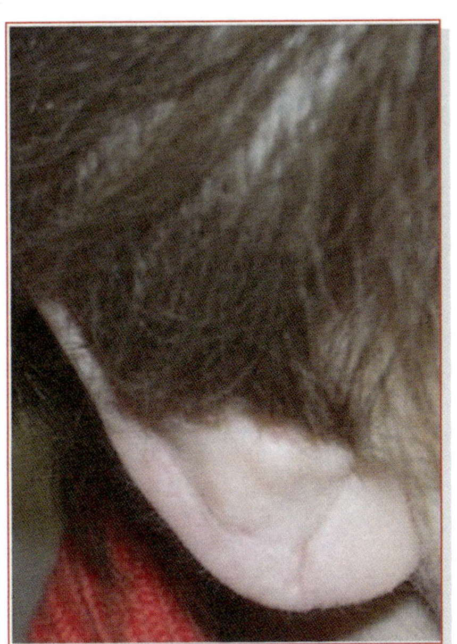
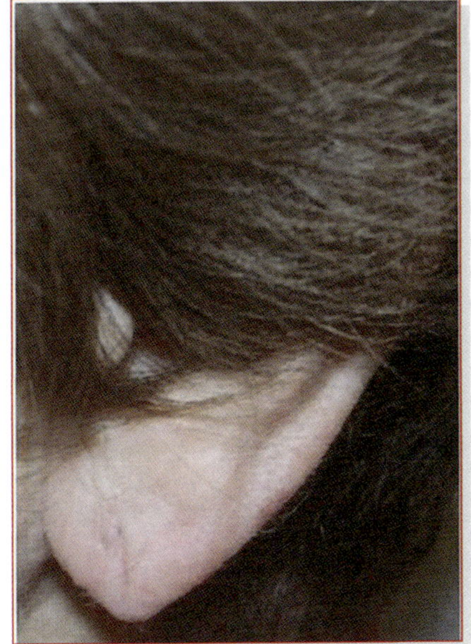

Final cosmetic result

Intense Pulsed Light

Intense pulsed light treats rosacea, lentigines (age spots and liver spots), and poikiloderma. Treatments use a very intense beam of light, which targets blood vessels and brown pigment. The rosacea, lentigines, and poikiloderma do not disappear immediately, but these conditions gradually fade. Some redness may be seen soon after sessions, but this calms down quickly. Sometimes additional treatments are needed to achieve further improvement, but it's best to wait a month before deciding if this is necessary. See the essay titled "Lentigo" in Part I of this book for some before and after photographs demonstrating the use of intense pulsed light for this condition.

PRETREATMENT DIRECTIONS

Patients treated for lentigines may apply lidocaine cream to the skin thirty minutes before sessions to reduce discomfort during treatment. LMX 4 and LMX 5 are brands of lidocaine cream available without a prescription. Patients treated for rosacea or poikiloderma should avoid lidocaine cream, which makes the treatment less effective.

POSTTREATMENT DIRECTIONS

Patients treated for lentigines or poikiloderma need to avoid too much sun exposure after sessions, or the condition could recur, reversing the benefits of the treatment. For advice on sun protection, see the beginning of the essay "Skin Aging: Prevention and Treatment" in Part I of this book.

Laser Hair Removal

Permanent hair removal using laser and intense pulsed light sources remains one of the most popular cosmetic procedures. These devices work by emitting light of a specific wavelength or band of wavelengths that targets brown pigment called melanin around the base of the hair shaft underneath the skin. When struck by light, the melanin and the hair's adjacent stem cells vaporize. Since melanin is the target of the device, hair without melanin, including blonde hair and white hair, responds poorly to treatment.

Approximately six treatments spaced at least one month apart are necessary to achieve complete, permanent hair removal, although fewer or more treatments may be necessary for any given patient. Why? Hairs progress through a life cycle, just like people. On any given day, only about 15 percent of hairs are in the part of the life cycle that makes them great targets for the laser. Therefore, after each treatment, approximately 15 percent of hairs will never come back, and approximately 85 percent of hairs will grow back. After six such treatments, the typical patient notices negligible hair regrowth.

PRETREATMENT DIRECTIONS

1. Avoid tanning before treatments. Tanned skin cannot be safely treated because it has lots of melanin in it—and the light emitted by the device cannot differentiate between melanin in tanned skin and melanin around the base of the hair shaft underneath the skin. Treating tanned skin could cause blistering and pigmentation changes. Therefore, avoiding excessive sun for six weeks before treatment and using sunscreen daily throughout the treatment course is recommended.

2. Avoid electrolysis, plucking, and waxing your hair for two weeks before treatment of facial hair, four weeks before treatment of

arm hair, and six weeks before leg hair. If you pluck or wax your hair prior to treatment, you have just removed the light's target, and the treatment won't work.

3. Please shave or clip your hair one day prior to treatment. Shaving and clipping will allow the light to penetrate better to the root of the hair without removing the light's target below. Bleaching your hair prior to treatment is also acceptable because it doesn't remove the roots' pigment.

4. If you have ever had fever blisters or cold sores in the treatment area, consider taking Valtrex (valacyclovir, 500 mg twice daily) beginning the day before treatment and continuing for two weeks after the treatment. Cold sores and fever blisters are caused by a herpes virus, and skin trauma from the procedure could cause the condition to recur.

5. Apply lidocaine cream to the treatment area thirty minutes before sessions to reduce discomfort. LMX 4 and LMX 5 are brands of lidocaine cream available without a prescription.

POSTTREATMENT DIRECTIONS

1. Post-treatment swelling and redness are usually minimal but could last a few days.

2. If scabs or crusts form, apply a moisturizer to the site until they resolve. Do not pick the scabs or crusts off.

3. Treated hairs may appear to grow for one to two weeks after treatment, but they will naturally fall out. Once inflammation has subsided, you can shave, tweeze, or wax these treated hairs. Hairs that have not been permanently vaporized during treatment may begin to grow two to six weeks after treatment.

Part III Cosmetic Treatments

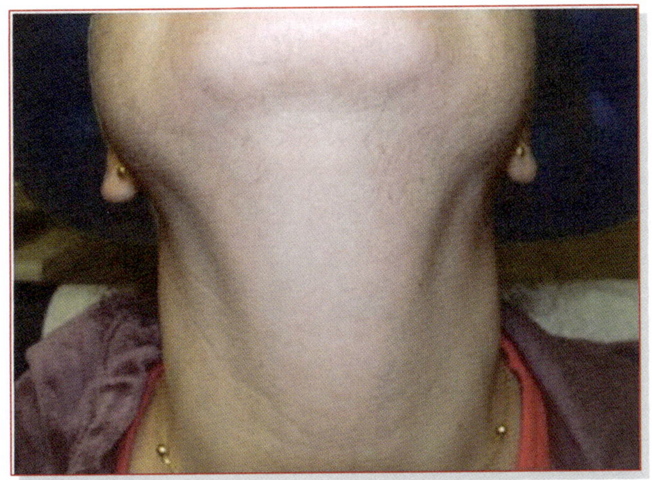

Before treatment with intense pulsed light

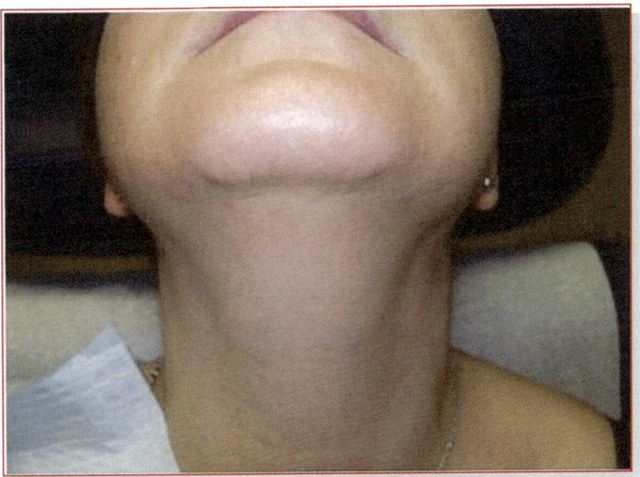

One month after the first treatment

Laser Resurfacing

Years of sunlight exposure leads to wrinkles, brown spots, and tiny blood vessels. These blemishes are all treatable with laser resurfacing. Successful treatment can take years off a person's appearance.

Recently, dermatologists have invented fractional resurfacing lasers that treat only a fraction of the skin per treatment session. These devices use a type of filter that allows only a fraction of the emitted laser light to reach the skin. Imagine light shining through a cheese grater that filters out 75 percent of the light.

Multiple treatment sessions spaced about one month apart may be required to achieve solid results with fractional resurfacing lasers. Patients often prefer this method because side effects are quite acceptable. For example, treatments typically leave the skin with a sunburned appearance for a few days, and if high settings are used, skin could peel for several days.

Patients looking for more dramatic results with fewer treatment sessions should consider traditional nonfractional, ablative laser resurfacing, which does not use a filter. This technique can leave your skin red and abraded-looking for a few weeks after treatment. Therefore, you should not expect to go back to work immediately after these sessions.

PRETREATMENT DIRECTIONS

1. Apply lidocaine cream to your skin thirty minutes before treatment to reduce discomfort. LMX 4 and LMX 5 are brands of lidocaine cream available without a prescription.

2. Patients undergoing fractional resurfacing on high settings and patients undergoing nonfractional, ablative laser resurfacing

should consider taking Valium (5 mg) forty-five minutes before treatment to reduce anxiety and discomfort. Tell your doctor if you want an anti-anxiety medicine. If you do take one, you will need a ride to and from the office.

3. To decrease discomfort and swelling, consider taking aspirin (325 mg) one hour before treatment and then every four hours for the rest of the day. Ask your doctor if this optional step is appropriate for you.

4. If you have ever had fever blisters or cold sores before, consider taking Valtrex (valacyclovir, 500 mg twice daily) beginning the day before resurfacing and continuing for two weeks after treatment. Cold sores and fever blisters are caused by a herpes virus, and skin trauma from the procedure could cause the condition to recur.

POSTTREATMENT DIRECTIONS

1. Apply a moisturizer, such as Aquaphor, until peeling is complete. If scabs or crusts form, apply a moisturizer to the site until they resolve. Do not pick the scabs or crusts off.

2. Consider using Cetaphil liquid cleanser as your soap. Patients can resume wearing makeup in a few days, when the skin has stopped peeling.

3. Limit your sun exposure to help prevent the recurrence of photo aging, actinic keratoses, fine wrinkles, and pigment irregularities that were treated. For advice on sun protection, see the beginning of the essay "Skin Aging: Prevention and Treatment" in Part I of this book.

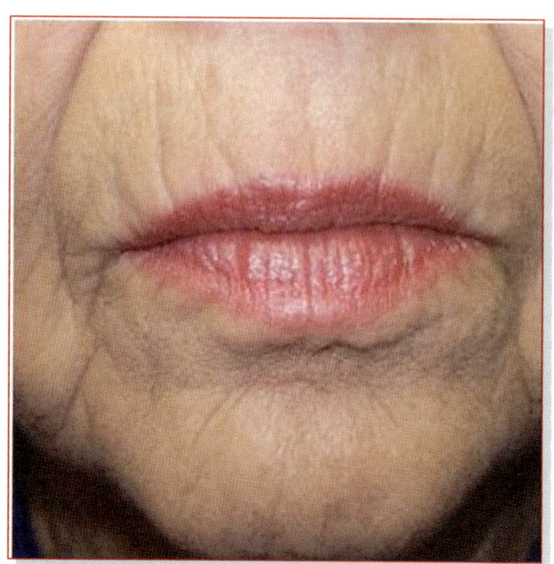

Before treatment of wrinkles around the lips

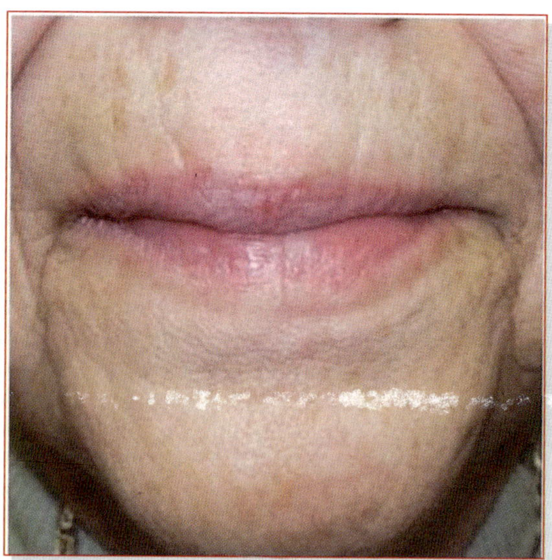

Improvement of wrinkles around the lips after fractional laser resurfacing

Laser Tattoo Removal

One of the great advances in laser medicine was the advent of quality-switched lasers for tattoo removal, creating a treatment that had been desired for centuries. According to Tina S. Alster, M.D., "Attempts at their removal date back to Egyptian mummies, who showed evidence of partial tattoo removal."[1] Quality-switched lasers emit light that targets tattoo pigment. Dermatologists hypothesize that when struck by laser light, shattered tattoo pigment is captured by immune cells and taken away via the lymphatic system.

PRETREATMENT DIRECTIONS

Six to twelve treatment sessions may be required to clear professional tattoos, but amateur tattoos may clear with fewer treatment sessions. Laser treatments are administered every four to eight weeks. Apply lidocaine cream thirty minutes before treatment to reduce discomfort. LMX 4 and LMX 5 are brands of lidocaine cream available without a prescription. Injections of lidocaine directly into the skin immediately prior to sessions may further reduce discomfort.

POSTTREATMENT DIRECTIONS

Swelling may last for three to five days, and bruising could last for one week. Apply an ice pack to reduce any bruising, swelling, and discomfort that could arise. Blistering or scabs may develop in the first days after treatment and will heal over faster if you apply a moisturizer, such as Aquaphor. Treated skin may also darken, especially in patients with darker complexions. Darkened skin fades over several months and may be prevented by avoiding excessive sun exposure. Finally, you could develop light-colored

---

[1]   Tina S. Alster, *Manual of Cutaneous Laser Techniques*, 2nd ed. (Philadelphia: Lippincott Williams and Wilkins; 2000), 71.

spots that resolve in several months, but there are rare cases in which they are permanent.

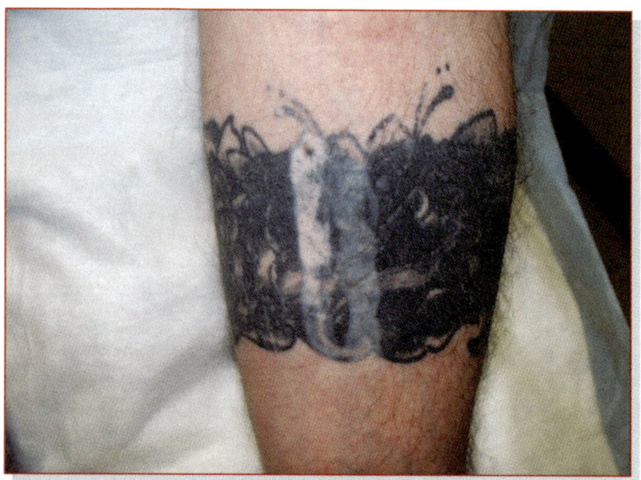

Significant lightening observed after a single test treatment of a professional black and green tattoo using a quality-switched Alexandrite laser. I passed the laser over the tattoo twice on the left side and once on the right side.

Part III Cosmetic Treatments

Radiesse

Radiesse is a filler designed to treat facial lines. As we age, our skin and the tissue underneath thin out—a process called atrophy. This creates lines on the face that are treatable with fillers. Radiesse is injected under the lines and rejuvenates a person's appearance by restoring this lost substance. It is FDA-approved for the treatment of facial lines, such as the two lines that run from the corners of the mouth to the bottom of the nose. Radiesse provides significant and noticeable improvement with a natural look. The filler is made of calcium hydroxylapatite, a natural substance that is broken down by the body into calcium and phosphorus. Results last approximately nine months.

PRETREATMENT DIRECTIONS

Swelling resolves in a matter of hours. Bruising is uncommon but may last up to a week. Please plan your social and work calendar accordingly. To reduce the likelihood of bruising, stop taking nonsteroidal anti-inflammatory medicines (ibuprofen or naprosyn), vitamin E, ginger, ginseng, ginkgo biloba, garlic, kava kava, celery root, and fish oils for one week prior to treatment. Do not stop aspirin if you have had a heart attack, stroke, or blood clot and are using it to prevent a recurrence. If you are taking aspirin for another reason, however, ask your doctor if you can stop taking it two weeks before the procedure. Finally, apply lidocaine cream to your skin thirty minutes before treatment to reduce discomfort. LMX 4 and LMX 5 are brands of lidocaine cream available without a prescription.

POSTTREATMENT DIRECTIONS

Apply an ice pack to reduce any swelling, redness, discomfort, or bruising that could arise. Also, take it easy when you go home— no heavy lifting or high-intensity exercise—but there are no other physical limitations for the day. Treat any lumpiness by massaging the area gently for five minutes every half hour.

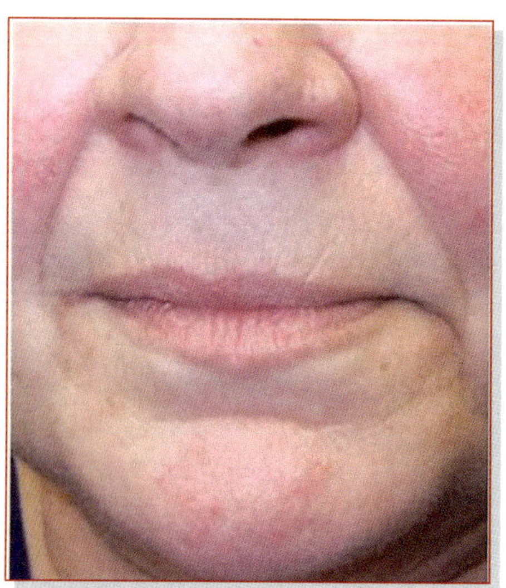

Lines before treatment with Radiesse

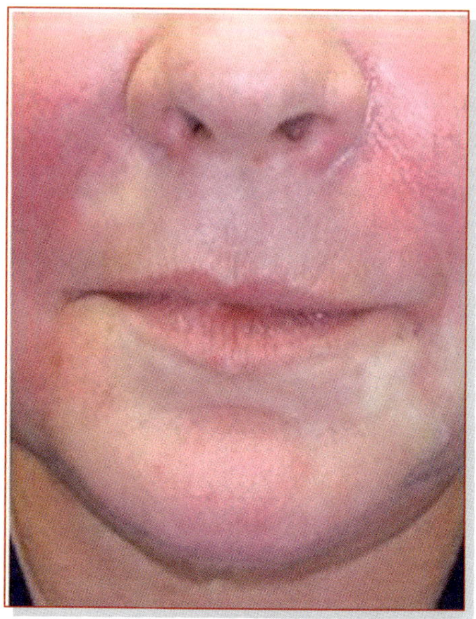

Immediately after treatment

Part III Cosmetic Treatments

Restylane and Juvederm

Juvederm and Restylane are fillers designed to treat facial lines. As we age, our skin and the tissue underneath thin out—a process called atrophy. This creates lines on the face that are treatable with fillers. Juvederm and Restylane are injected under the lines and help eliminate them by restoring this lost substance. They are most often used for the two lines that run from the corners of the mouth to the bottom of the nose. The dermatologist may also inject these fillers into the lips or under sunken lower eyelids to provide additional volume where needed. Juvederm and Restylane provide significant and noticeable improvement with a natural look. These fillers are made of hyaluronic acid, a sugar-like substance found naturally in the body. After injections, your body slowly breaks down the material, and results typically last six months.

PRETREATMENT DIRECTIONS

Swelling typically resolves in a matter of hours. Bruising is uncommon but may last up to a week if it occurs. Please plan your social and work calendar accordingly. To decrease the likelihood of bruising, stop taking nonsteroidal anti-inflammatory medicines (ibuprofen or naprosyn), vitamin E, ginger, ginseng, ginkgo biloba, garlic, kava kava, celery root, and fish oils for one week prior to the procedure. Do not stop aspirin if you have had a heart attack, stroke, or blood clot and are using it to prevent a recurrence. If you are taking aspirin for another reason, however, ask your doctor if you can stop taking it two weeks before the procedure. Finally, apply lidocaine cream to your skin thirty minutes before treatment to reduce discomfort. LMX 4 and LMX 5 are brands of lidocaine cream available without a prescription.

POSTTREATMENT DIRECTIONS

Apply an ice pack to reduce any swelling, redness, discomfort, or bruising that could arise. Also, take it easy when you go home—no heavy lifting or high-intensity exercise—but there are no other physical limitations for the day. Treat any lumpiness by massaging the area gently for five minutes every half hour.

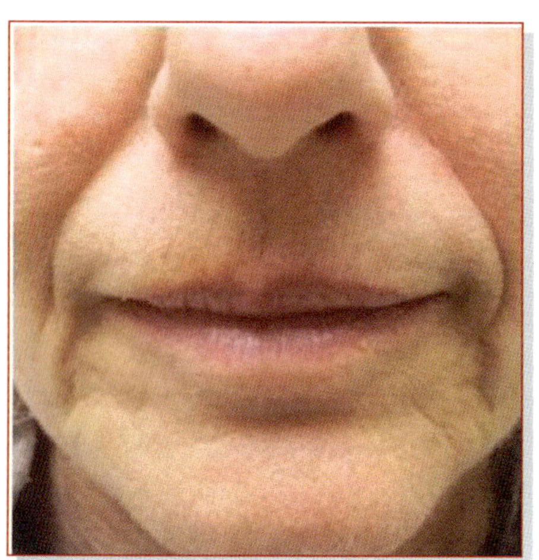

Lines before treatment

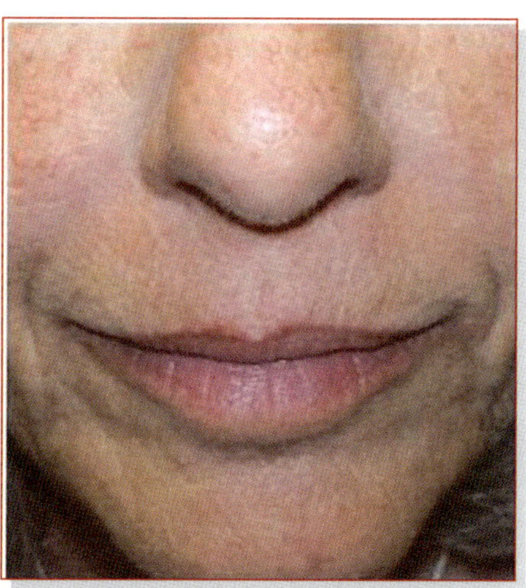

Cosmetic result after treatment with Juvederm

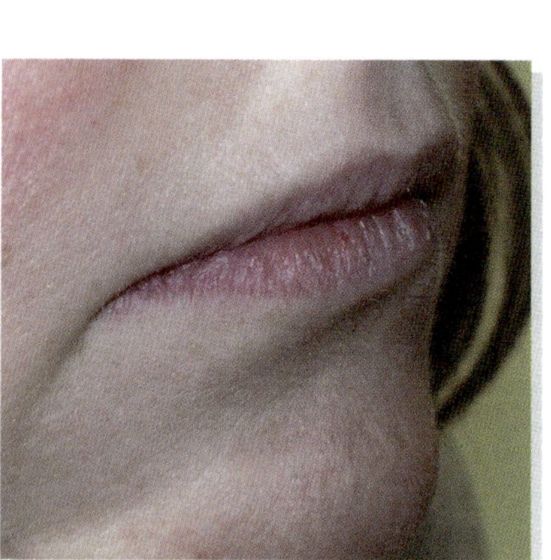

Lips before treatment

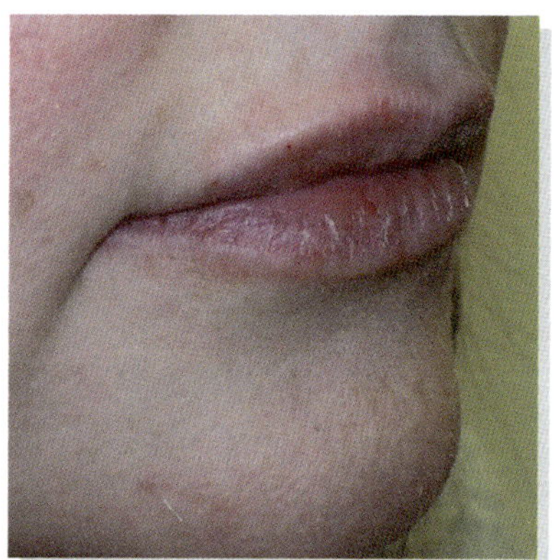

Lips after treatment with Juvederm

Sclerotherapy

Sclerotherapy treats tiny blue leg veins, also called reticular veins or venulectasias. This condition may arise in adulthood due to a decline in function of deeper, non-visible veins, which return blood from the feet back to the heart. When these deep vessels stop working, blood backs up in them, and smaller reticular veins and venulectasias become enlarged and visible.

Sclerotherapy is performed by injecting a sclerosant, such as a concentrated salt solution, into the vessels, causing them to collapse. Best results are obtained if compression stockings are worn for three weeks after treatment. Put them on in the morning and remove them at night. The Jobst brand of compression stockings may be purchased without a prescription at surgical supply stores and local and online pharmacies. Only a percentage of vessels disappear permanently after any given treatment session, and two to five treatment sessions may be required at six- to eight-week intervals to achieve satisfactory results.

Sclerotherapy is generally well tolerated, but some people develop pain or cramping at the injection sites. Others may develop temporary dark patches at the site of injections. Finally, skin sloughing has been reported, though uncommonly.

The appearance of tiny vessels on your legs may warrant a search for broken deeper, non-visible veins with a duplex Doppler ultrasound test. This test may be needed if you suffer from leg swelling or pain. Vein specialists may remove broken deeper veins or treat them with a laser.

Part IV
Surgical and Other Treatments and Tests

Biopsy

In an ideal world, a dermatologist would be able to glance at your skin and know exactly what you have. The real world works differently. In many cases, the dermatologist may not be absolutely sure what condition you have and need more information to figure it out. A biopsy is a procedure designed to provide the additional needed information.

Please don't worry. Most biopsies are easier than a dental cleaning, and in 99 percent of cases, patients report it was a much better experience than they originally feared. It takes about five minutes to perform a biopsy.

First, the dermatologist injects some lidocaine into the area to numb the skin. You feel some pinching and stinging during this part, but it goes away rapidly. Lidocaine works amazingly fast; in my opinion, whoever invented it deserves the Nobel Prize.

You will not feel anything uncomfortable as the biopsy proceeds. When trying to rule out skin cancer, dermatologists often perform a shave biopsy by literally shaving off a piece of skin with a blade. The specimen is placed in a cup and sent to the pathologist, and the remaining small wound is covered with a bandage. Finally, you need to perform daily dressing changes at home until the site heals over.

A shave biopsy is not always appropriate. When trying to determine the cause of a rash, dermatologists often perform a punch biopsy with an instrument called a punch tool that removes a tiny, cylindrical piece of skin. The specimen is placed in a cup and sent to the pathologist. Sutures close the biopsy site, which is then covered with a bandage. You will need to perform daily dressing changes at home and return to the office for suture removal in one to two weeks.

Pathologists usually deliver their results within a week. Call your dermatologist if you have not received your results within two weeks after the biopsy.

Highlights of a Punch Biopsy

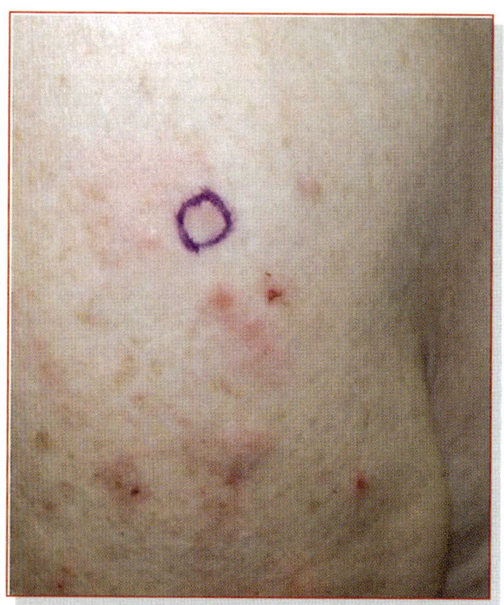

The dermatologist demarcates the planned biopsy site with a marking pen.

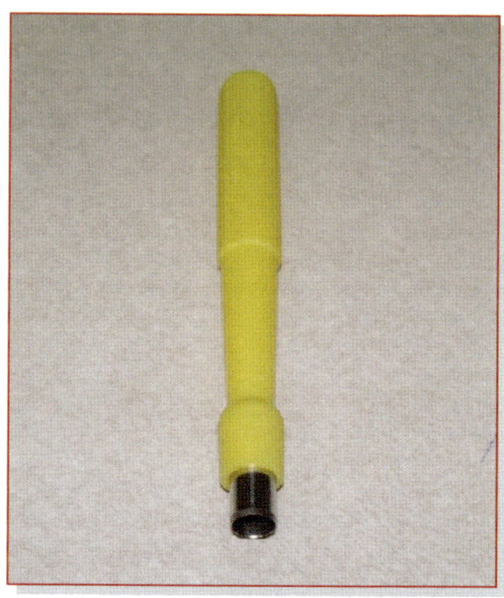

Punch tool

The dermatologist sends the punched-out skin for pathology examination.

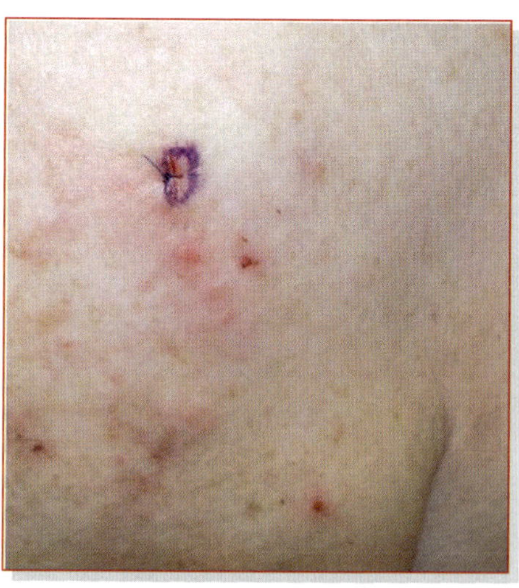

The dermatologist closes the biopsy site with a suture.

Part IV Surgical and Other Treatments and Tests

Skin Care Instructions for After a Biopsy

DAY OF THE BIOPSY

Keep the dressing on your biopsy site dry and protected.

INSTRUCTIONS FOR ALL SUBSEQUENT DAYS UNTIL YOU RETURN FOR SUTURE REMOVAL OR UNTIL THE SHAVE BIOPSY SITE HEALS OVER COMPLETELY

Wet the dressing daily in the shower and gently remove it. Then cleanse the biopsy site with soap and water, hydrogen peroxide, white vinegar (one tablespoon in one pint of water), or Hibiclens (chlorhexidine). Hibiclens is available without a prescription at local and online pharmacies. If using Hibiclens, do not get any in your eyes or ears. Use only soap and water close to the eyes. Then apply Vaseline or other ointment, such as mupirocin, Neosporin, Polysporin, or Bacitracin, to the biopsy site with a Q-tip. Finally, apply an adhesive bandage to keep the site protected.

SPECIAL DIRECTIONS

1. If the dressing gets wet or falls off, replace it as described above.

2. If you develop a red, itchy rash at the biopsy site, you may be developing a skin allergy to the antibiotic ointment or bandage. Consider stopping use of the antibiotic ointment and using Vaseline only, which will not cause skin allergies.

3. If you develop pain, redness, swelling, warmth, pus, or a foul odor at the biopsy site, you may be developing an infection. Call your doctor because you may need oral antibiotics.

4. If you bleed through the bandage, fold up some first-aid gauze
   pads and apply them firmly to the biopsy site for twenty minutes. If the site is still bleeding, repeat the firm application
   of folded gauze for another twenty minutes. If the site is still
   bleeding after the second application, call your doctor or go to
   the emergency room.

5. If you have not received your results within two weeks, call your
   dermatologist.

Excision

Dermatologists perform excisions to definitively remove a skin growth. They are often performed after a biopsy has already confirmed the existence of a skin cancer, but excisions may also be performed to remove a cyst or lipoma without a preceding biopsy. The procedure takes approximately forty-five minutes, and it isn't very difficult or painful. Afterward, most patients report it was easier than going to the dentist.

First, the dermatologist injects some lidocaine around the growth to numb the area. You feel some pinching and stinging, but that rapidly dissipates. Then, the dermatologist removes the growth and a small moat of normal looking skin around it with a scalpel. You do not feel this part of the procedure. The shape of the moat is usually elliptical, not circular, in order to allow the skin edges to come together in a flat, pleasing fashion.

The dermatologist then places sutures to pull the edges of the skin together. Absorbable sutures are placed underneath the skin, and they will dissolve with time. A second layer of non-absorbable sutures is placed on the skin surface, and these sutures are typically removed in two weeks.

The skin specimen is sent to the pathologist to confirm what the lesion is and, if cancer, to confirm that it has been entirely removed. Pathologists usually deliver their results within a week. Call your dermatologist if you have not received your results within two weeks.

Highlights of an Excision

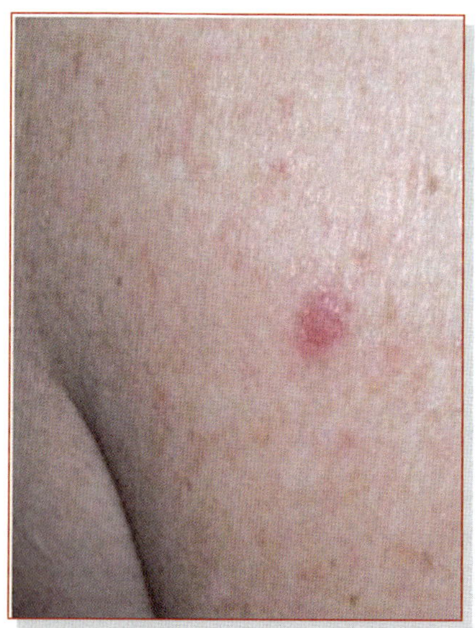

Basal cell carcinoma on the right arm.

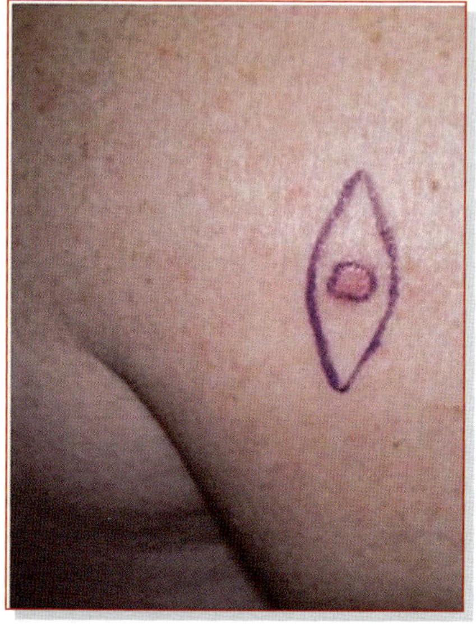

The dermatologist draws an elliptical-shaped moat around the skin cancer.

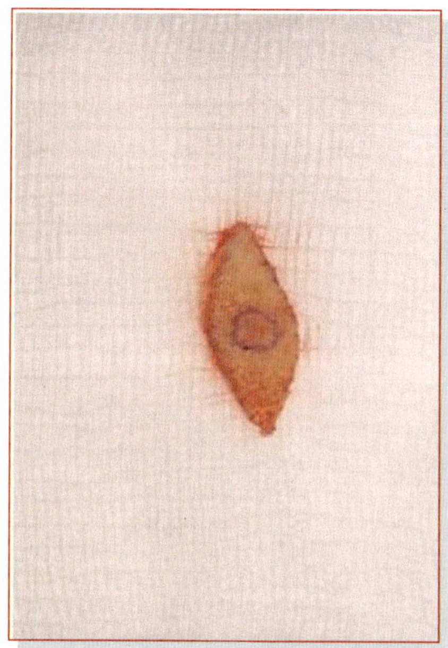

Excised tissue is sent to the pathologist.

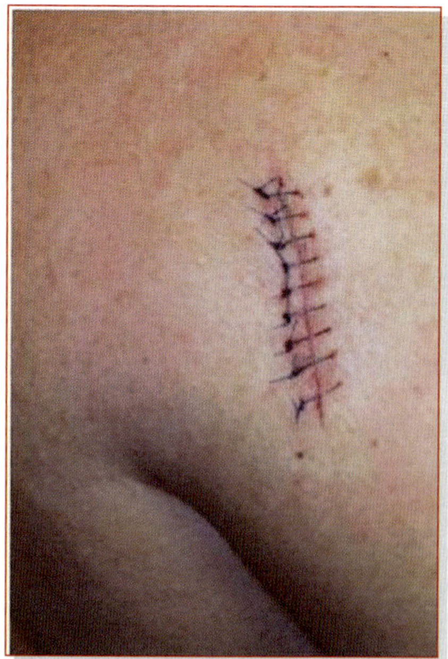

The surgical site is closed with sutures.

Mohs Micrographic Surgery

Mohs micrographic surgery is a technique used for removing skin cancers. It was invented by Dr. Frederic E. Mohs at the University of Wisconsin. Over the past several decades, the procedure has undergone continued evolution and is now considered the treatment of choice for the most common skin cancers under certain conditions.

Mohs surgery is performed in the office with a local anesthetic—you do not have to go to the operating room, and you will not be asleep for the procedure. The surgery is performed in stages. In the first stage, the surgeon injects some lidocaine around the growth to numb the area. You feel some pinching and stinging, but that rapidly dissipates. The surgeon then removes the skin cancer and a small margin of normal-looking skin around it with a scalpel. You do not feel this part of the procedure. The removed skin is processed in the office and analyzed under a microscope by the same surgeon. If microscopic analysis shows that the skin cancer has been removed completely, the surgical site is then bandaged over and allowed to heal in or is repaired with plastic surgery techniques. Sometimes, however, microscopic analysis shows that the skin cancer is not all out, in which case additional skin is removed. In this second stage, the skin is again processed and analyzed under the microscope. The procedure continues in this fashion until the skin cancer is removed completely, at which point the surgical site is repaired with sutures or is bandaged over and allowed to heal in on its own. The average number of stages required for Mohs surgery is two, and the average stage takes twenty-five minutes, but the number of stages per case and the average time per stage can vary widely. Time required for sewing up the surgical site can vary greatly, too, depending upon the complexity of the case.

Cure rates for Mohs surgery are high compared with the alternatives. Published five-year cure rates for the treatment of a primary basal cell carcinoma are 99 percent, and published five-year cure rates for a primary squamous cell carcinoma are 97 percent.

These results exceed those achievable with radiation therapy, excision, liquid nitrogen, and electrodessication and curettage.[2]

Doctors master Mohs surgery and the art of surgical reconstruction during a one-year fellowship offered by the American College of Mohs Surgery. This fellowship is typically completed after a residency in dermatology. For best results, find a Mohs surgeon who has completed this one-year fellowship.

PREOPERATIVE DIRECTIONS

1. Bring your spouse or another trusted person on the day of the procedure. He or she may be needed to confirm the site of the skin cancer. In addition, he or she may provide a second set of ears as the medical staff provides you with many instructions.

2. On the day of your surgery, eat regular meals beforehand.

3. Do not discontinue blood thinners if they have been prescribed by your physician, especially if you have had a heart attack, stroke, or blood clot. Aspirin, Coumadin (warfarin), Plavix (clopidogrel), and Pradaxa (dabigatran) are common blood thinners. If you have never had a heart attack, stroke, or blood clot, and you are taking aspirin for other reasons, you may consider stopping it two weeks before surgery and restarting it two weeks after surgery. Ask your doctor if this is acceptable in your case before making a decision.

4. Nonsteroidal anti-inflammatory medicines commonly used for headaches and joint pain may increase your risk for bleeding. These medicines include Advil or Motrin (ibuprofen), Aleve or Naprosyn (naproxen), Arthrotec (diclofenac), Indocin (indomethacin), Mobic (meloxicam), and Clinoril (sulindac). If you have a normally functioning liver, Tylenol is a preferred pain medicine that will not increase your risk for bleeding. Other supplements that may increase

---

[2] Stephen N. Snow and George R. Mikhail, ed., Mohs Micrographic Surgery, 2nd ed. (Madison: University of Wisconsin Press, 2005), 45.

your risk for bleeding include fish oil, garlic, ginkgo biloba, glucosamine, and vitamin E. Please avoid these supplements for up to two weeks before the procedure and one week after the procedure.

5. Shower before the procedure, and wear freshly cleaned but informal clothes the day of the procedure. If the surgery site is above your waist, wear a very loose-fitting shirt or sweatshirt that easily and quickly comes off and on. Do not wear a formal button-down shirt. If the surgery site is below your waist, wear shorts or very loose-fitting sweatpants that quickly come off and on. Moreover, if the surgery is on your foot, bring footwear that could easily fit over a bulky dressing. After the surgery, while your surgical site is healing, continue to wear freshly cleaned clothes. Keeping clean will help prevent infections.

6. Do not wear jewelry or apply creams, makeup, or aftershave lotions near the surgery site on the day of your procedure and the day you return for suture removal.

7. Bring something to snack on and something to read during the procedure because you may spend many hours at the office.

8. If the surgery site is around your eyes, the bandage may affect your ability to wear glasses, making driving home difficult. Arrange for a safe ride home under these circumstances.

9. Inform your doctor if you have had any of the following: trouble stopping bleeding in the past, serious skin infection by *Staphylococcus aureus,* an artificial heart valve, artificial joint, pacemaker, or defibrillator. Also inform your doctor if you have a heart murmur or if you take antibiotics before dental procedures.

10. Many patients feel much calmer if they have taken Valium (5 mg) immediately before the procedure. Valium reduces stress and anxiety. Tell the surgeon if you wish to take an anti-anxiety medicine. You will need a ride to and from the office if you take this medication.

Highlights of a Mohs Surgery

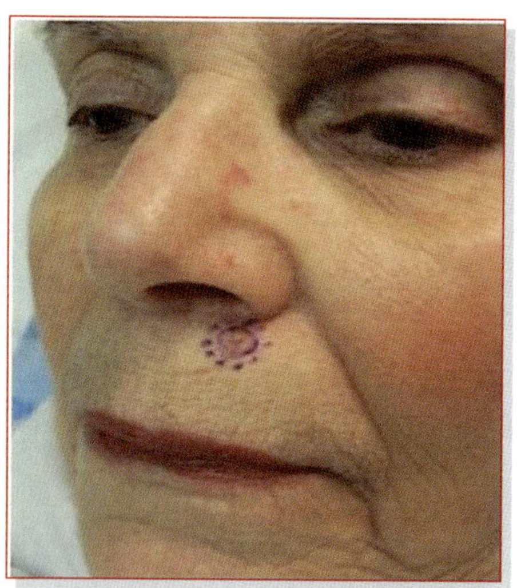

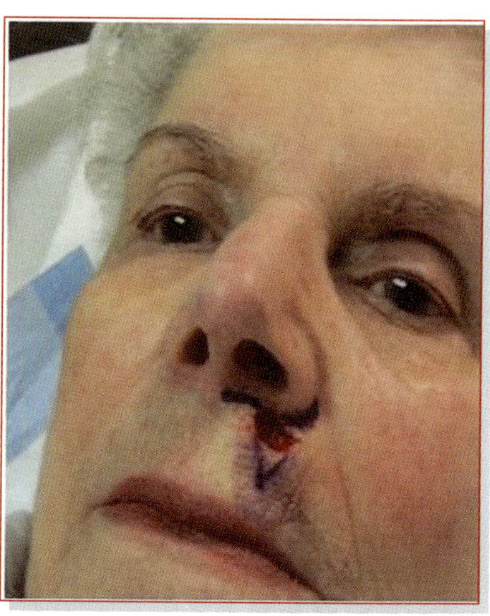

The surgeon demarcates a basal cell carcinoma with a marking pen. During the first stage of surgery, he removes all the skin within the dots. It pops out in the shape of a dime.

The surgeon excised the basal cell carcinoma. Histology demonstrated its complete removal. Finally, he designs an advancement flap with a marking pen to repair the surgical site.

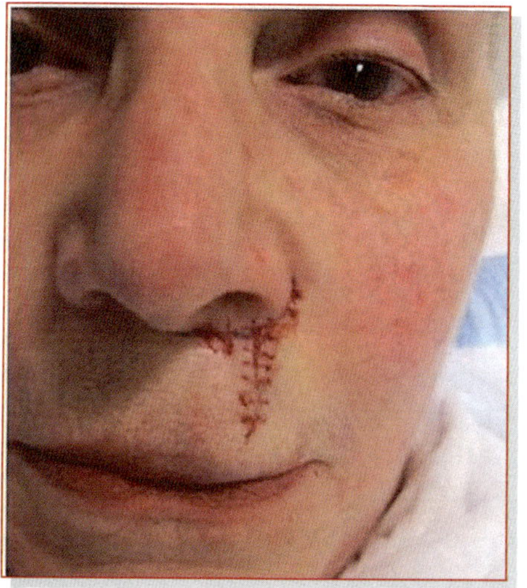

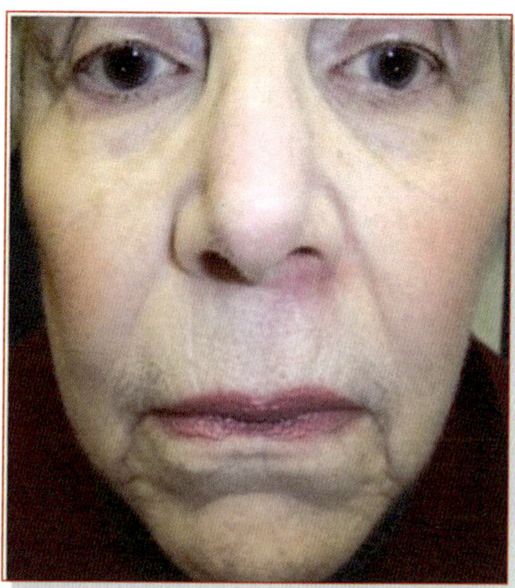

The surgeon places the flap to close the surgical site.

Final cosmetic result.

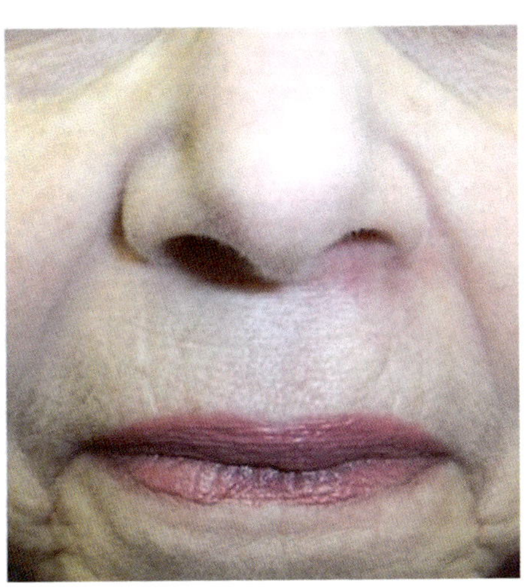

Close-up of the cosmetic result.

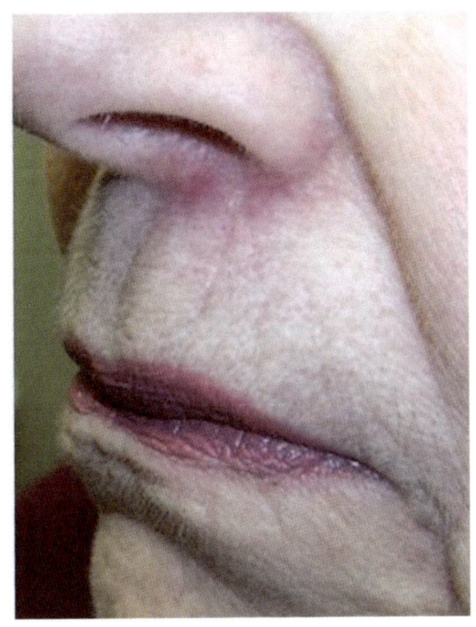

Close-up of the cosmetic result.

Skin Care Instructions for After an Excision or Mohs Surgery

DAY OF THE EXCISION OR MOHS SURGERY

Keep the surgical site dry and protected.

INSTRUCTIONS FOR ALL SUBSEQUENT DAYS UNTIL YOU RETURN TO THE OFFICE

Soak the dressing in the shower and gently remove the dressing after washing your hands. Cleanse the surgical site with one of the following: hydrogen peroxide, white vinegar (one tablespoon in one pint of water), or Hibiclens (chlorhexidine) using fresh gauze or Q-tips. Hibiclens is available without a prescription at local and online pharmacies. If using Hibiclens, do not get it in your eyes or ears. Hydrogen peroxide works particularly well to dissolve any crusts that have formed around the surgical site, but please do not forcefully pick off any adherent crusts—this could cause bleeding. Finally, use only soap and water close to the eyes.

Apply Vaseline or other ointment, such as mupirocin, Bacitracin, Polysporin, or Neosporin, to the surgical site with a Q-tip. Keep your surgical site moist because moist wounds heal significantly faster than dry wounds. Finally, apply a two-layer dressing by placing a nonstick pad directly to the skin, and then cover this pad with first-aid gauze. Telfa is a brand of nonstick pad commonly used in dermatology clinics. Finally, secure the dressing with first-aid cloth tape. If the surgical site is small enough, and nothing is draining from it, you may apply a large adhesive bandage over the wound instead of a two-layer dressing.

SPECIAL DIRECTIONS

1. Do not smoke when you go home until wound healing is complete. Smoking deprives the surgical site of oxygen, which is needed for healing.

2. Apply an ice pack as time allows to reduce discomfort, swelling, bleeding, and bruising.

3. If you have a normally functioning liver, Tylenol is typically preferred for postoperative discomfort because other pain medicines increase the risk for bleeding. Most patients with a healthy liver and kidneys can take up to two extra-strength Tylenol every four hours, as needed. Consider taking Tylenol upon arriving home, even before the numbing medicine wears off.

4. If the dressing gets wet or falls off, replace it as described above.

5. If you bleed through your bandage, fold up some first-aid gauze pads and press them firmly onto the surgical site for twenty minutes. After twenty minutes, check the wound. If it is still bleeding, repeat the firm application of gauze for another twenty minutes. If the site is still bleeding after the second application, call your surgeon or go to the closest emergency room.

6. If you develop severe pain or swelling around the surgery site, you could be developing a hematoma, which is a collection of blood under the skin. Please call your surgeon promptly because you may need treatment.

7. If you develop a red, itchy rash at the surgery site, you may be developing a skin allergy to the antibiotic ointment or dressing.

Consider stopping the use of antibiotic ointment and use Vaseline only, which will not cause a skin allergy.

8. If you develop pain, redness, swelling, warmth, pus, or foul odor at the surgery site, you could have an infection. Call your surgeon because you may need oral antibiotics.

9. If the surgery was on your face or head, try to keep your head elevated for the next forty-eight hours. Bending down causes blood to rush to your head and may increase the likelihood of bleeding. Also, elevate your head on two to three pillows at night if possible.

10. If the surgery was below your knee, expect some redness and swelling to persist for several weeks. You can reduce redness and swelling by elevating your legs when sitting. A seat cane, available at surgical supply stores, may be useful for this purpose, especially when you plan to leave your house. Ice packs will also reduce discomfort, redness, and swelling. Finally, excessive walking and standing increase pain, redness, and swelling, so please take it easy.

11. If the surgery was around your mouth, eat only soft foods (for example, rice, yogurt, apple sauce, and so forth) for three days after the procedure. Opening your mouth too wide or stretching your lips while eating something large or firm can cause bleeding.

12. Avoid strenuous exercise for approximately three weeks after the procedure. Activities that increase your pulse or blood pressure could cause bleeding or pull apart your stitches.

13. Wear only clean clothes over the surgery site to decrease the risk for infection.

   Part IV Surgical and Other Treatments and Tests

14. If the surgical site was left to heal from the inside out without sutures, you must cleanse the wound and change the dressing daily until the site is completely healed over. Healed wounds are pink and smooth. They are not covered with scabs, and they do not leak fluid. Most wounds require a few weeks to heal, but wounds below the knees may take significantly longer because circulation in this area is relatively poor. Finally, the scar may appear light-colored compared with surrounding skin.

15. Surgical scars tend to look increasingly better over the course of an entire year, even with no treatment. Nevertheless, after suture removal, you may consider treating the scar to improve its appearance. For example, massaging the scar with your fingers periodically throughout the day for several months may help soften and flatten the scar. Silicone sheets also soften and flatten scars. These sheets are available at pharmacies and are taped to the scar at night and removed in the morning. Use them for four to six months for best results.

    If the scar's color bothers you, a pulsed dye laser can remove the pink color. Dermatologists can also treat puffy scars with corticosteroid injections, which help them settle down. Finally, the doctor can polish your scar with a procedure called dermabrasion.

Patch Testing for Allergic Contact Dermatitis

Allergic contact dermatitis presents as an itchy pink rash. Patch testing helps identify the chemical that could be causing it and requires three office visits. Do not apply any corticosteroid creams to your back for two weeks prior to your patch test placement.

OFFICE VISIT 1

The dermatologist tapes eight paper patches onto your back. These patches contain eighty different chemicals that commonly cause allergic contact dermatitis. Wear loose-fitting clothing on this day, because tight-fitting clothes may rub the patches off your back. Also, do not apply any creams to your back on this day because creams will prevent the patches from sticking to your skin.

You may develop itching under the patches, which may be a sign that you are allergic to one of the test chemicals. Do not scratch the patches since this can shift them and make interpretation of results difficult.

Keep your back dry at home. Getting your back wet may cause the patches to fall off. Therefore, instead of showering, keep clean by washing with a sponge. Also, avoid heavy lifting, excessive bending, and physical and aerobic exercises that could cause sweating and detachment of the patches.

Wear loose-fitting clothing at home and a T-shirt in bed to prevent the patches from peeling off. If the patches start peeling off, pressure the adhesive back onto your skin or apply additional tape.

OFFICE VISIT 2

Two days later the dermatologist removes your patches and notes all skin reactions. He or she then applies a felt-tipped pen to the skin to specify exactly where the patches were initially placed. Wear an old T-shirt on this day because the marking pen could wipe off your back onto clothing. When you go home, avoid showering and exercising because moisture on your back could wipe off the marking pen. Wash with a sponge as before.

OFFICE VISIT 3

Two to five days later, the dermatologist examines your back for any delayed skin reactions. The doctor then discusses what is causing your rash and recommends using or avoiding specific products, depending on the results.

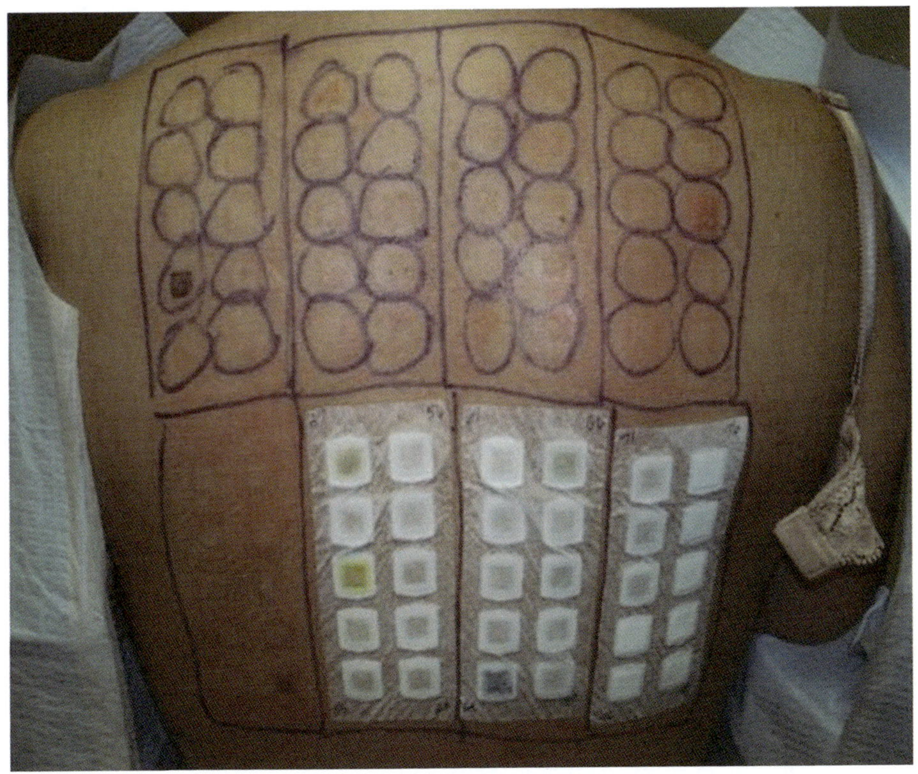

During office visit 2, some patches were removed and markings placed to specify where each chemical had been exposed to the skin.

Wet Dressing

Many skin conditions, such as eczema, cause extreme itching. The application of wet dressings is a safe and effective way to reduce itching and inflammation in the skin. You will need a corticosteroid cream and a 100 percent cotton dressing to cover the affected skin. Long underwear, T-shirts, pajamas, socks, gloves, bath towels, and cloth diapers are examples of dressings typically utilized.

DIRECTIONS

1. Waterproof a chair or bed with large plastic garbage bags cut into large sheets. Then cover the plastic with a bed sheet or large bath towel, and turn up the heat in the room so you won't get cold during treatment.

2. Place the cotton dressings (e.g. socks if the rash is on your feet) in a basin filled with warm water, then squeeze them out so they are wet but not dripping.

3. Apply the corticosteroid cream to your skin then the wet dressing over the affected area. Cover the wet dressings with dry towels or a sweat suit.

4. Sit or lie on the waterproofed chair or bed for thirty to sixty minutes.

5. Remove all the coverings and apply a moisturizer, such as Cetaphil, to your skin.

6. Wash and dry your dressings.

7. Apply wet dressings up to three times a day as needed.